Advances in Human Vector Control

ACS SYMPOSIUM SERIES **1014**

Advances in Human Vector Control

J. Marshall Clark, Editor
University of Massachusetts

Jeffrey R. Bloomquist, Editor
Virginia Polytechnic Institute and State Universtiy

Hitoshi Kawada, Editor
Nagasaki University

Sponsored by the
ACS AGRO Division
Pesticide Science Society of Japan

American Chemical Society, Washington DC

Library of Congress Cataloging-in-Publication Data

Advances in human vector control / J. Marshall Clark, editor ; sponsored by the ACS AGRO Division, Pesticide Science Society of Japan.
p. ; cm. -- (ACS symposium series ; 1014)
Includes bibliographical references and indexes.
ISBN 978-0-8412-6977-4 (alk. paper)
1. Vector control. 2. Insects--Control. 3. Insects as carriers of disease. 4. Insecticides. I. Clark, J. Marshall (John Marshall), 1949- II. American Chemical Society. Division of Agrochemicals. III. American Chemical Society. IV. Nihon Noyaku Gakkai. V. Series: ACS symposium series, 1014. 0097-6156 ;
[DNLM: 1. Insect Control--methods. 2. Arachnid Vectors. 3. Insect Vectors. 4. Insecticides. 5. Pest Control. QX 600 A2435 2009]

RA639.3.A38 2009
614.4'3--dc22

2009020530

The paper used in this publication meets the minimum requirements of American National Standard for Information Sciences—Permanence of Paper for Printed Library Materials, ANSI Z39.48–1984.

Distributed by Oxford University Press

PRINTED IN THE UNITED STATES OF AMERICA

Foreword

The ACS Symposium Series was first published in 1974 to provide a mechanism for publishing symposia quickly in book form. The purpose of the series is to publish timely, comprehensive books developed from the ACS sponsored symposia based on current scientific research. Occasionally, books are developed from symposia sponsored by other organizations when the topic is of keen interest to the chemistry audience.

Before agreeing to publish a book, the proposed table of contents is reviewed for appropriate and comprehensive coverage and for interest to the audience. Some papers may be excluded to better focus the book; others may be added to provide comprehensiveness. When appropriate, overview or introductory chapters are added. Drafts of chapters are peer-reviewed prior to final acceptance or rejection, and manuscripts are prepared in camera-ready format.

As a rule, only original research papers and original review papers are included in the volumes. Verbatim reproductions of previous published papers are not accepted.

ACS Books Department

Contents

Introduction

Current Status and Control Practices

Novel Approaches and Resistance Management

Indexes

Introduction

Chapter 1

Vector Biology Diagnostics and Public Health Pesticide Development through the Product Development Partnership Route.

Janet Hemingway

Liverpool School of Tropical Medicine, Pembroke Place, Liverpool L3 5QA, UK
Email hemingway@liv.ac.uk

Public Health Pesticides play a key role in the control of many insect vector borne diseases. These include diseases causing severe human morbidity and mortality, such as malaria, dengue, filariasis, Japanese encephalitis and West Nile. The largest volume of insecticide is used to contain malaria, which still afflicts much of the tropical and sub-tropical world.

Malaria elimination was attempted in the 1960s on the back of the discovery and deployment of DDT to control the mosquito vectors and chloroquine to control the parasite infections. Failure of the campaign has often been linked to the appearance of DDT resistance in many of the mosquito vectors, although the lack of political will to maintain the funding, infrastructure and vertical programmes needed for a sustained elimination campaign were probably more relevant. While the campaign failed to achieve its major objectives, the many successes in this early elimination campaign served to underline the make or break role that vector control has both in elimination and sustained control campaigns in areas of high and moderate malaria transmission. It is the lead intervention in the current Global Malaria Action Plan and the only tool that is capable of bringing intense or moderate transmission down to the low levels where elimination supported by drug treatment and vaccination is within reach. However, insecticides, like drugs and antibiotics have a finite product lifespan.

The average lifespan of an agrochemical insecticide is approximately 40 years. The longevity of the product is heavily influenced by its efficacy compared to competitor products, the ability of the manufacturer to maintain its licenses to sell in an increasingly complex regulatory environment, and the rate at which the target insects against which it is used become operationally resistant. The market operates well where the market size and net profitability of the product, over the time period over which patent rights reduce generic competition, are sufficient to generate a substantive return once the capital costs associated with insecticide production plant, development, manufacture and sales costs have been factored into the calculations. Market size and profit margins within the high volume, low margin, tender-based public health pesticide market for malaria and most other vector borne diseases are not sufficiently large to stimulate industry to develop and maintain a robust pipeline of new Public Health Insecticides. All previous Public Health Pesticides were developed as formulations of existing agrochemical insecticides. While this generated four classes of public health insecticides for operational vector control over four decades trends of increasing selectivity and the move away from contact toxicity to delivery systemically through the crop plant, have meant that newer classes of agrochemicals cannot easily be repurposed for public health use. It is not surprising therefore, that DDT, despite its obvious environmental issues has still been retained for malaria control because of the severely restricted range of available alternatives.

Over 20 publicly or charitably funded Product Development Partnerships (PDPs) now exist to share the risk and cost of developing a large range of drugs, vaccines and diagnostics for ‘orphan’ diseases whose market size and value would not warrant individual company investment. These have rejuvenated the R & D activities of the pharmaceutical industry for a range of diseases. The issues around Public Health Pesticides are very similar to those for ‘orphan’ drugs, with the baseline costs of ~US$200Million per new insecticide developed being prohibitive for the agrochemical industry alone to underwrite using normal industrial risk assessments and NPV calculations. The net result of this has been the long term disengagement of the agrochemical industry from development of new compounds into the public health market with a concomitant deskilling of industry in this area. The Innovative Vector Control Consortium (IVCC) is the first PDP established to work with the agrochemical industry to redress this imbalance, by providing access to funding and expertise to stimulate the industry to re-engage [1].

Indoor residual spraying (IRS) was developed to routinely bring DDT into contact with the adult female mosquitoes at the most epidemiologically significant point of contact between man and insect. Insecticide impregnated bednets (ITNs) followed in the 1980s, breaking man-mosquito contact for night biting insects and providing both community and personal protection for the users. Long-lasting ITNs (LLINs) were developed in the 1990s using technology to ensure that the insecticide remained on the net for the useful life of the net itself. There has been little innovation in effective treatments since then, despite the seriousness of the health problem. Coils, impregnated mats for emanators and aerosols are readily available in the consumer markets, but there is little direct evidence for these impacting on disease transmission and the annual cost of routinely using these interventions is high despite the low cost of the individual coils or sprays.

Establishing whether Public Health Pesticides, presented in different formats to control the vector population, can effectively control disease is non-trivial, as is monitoring the effectiveness of current control campaigns. Data on parasite infection rates in humans and insects, insect population density, insecticide coverage rates, effectiveness of treatment, climate and geography need to be efficiently collected and analysed to make the link between disease in man, parasite transmission and interventions affecting the mosquito's biology and ecology. This data has usually to be collected from very remote areas in very resource poor settings.

The Innovative Vector Control Consortium (IVCC) was established in November 2005 with an initial US$50.7M investment from the Bill and Melinda Gates Foundation, to start and address a number of these issues. The initial investment leveraged further funding from the Wellcome Trust (UK), National Institutes of Health, USA and European Union to expand the scope of some of the original diagnostics work. The IVCC was instigated with two separate arms. The first developing better diagnostics and software systems to allow control programmes to monitor and evaluate their vector control interventions, both programmatically and experimentally. The second arm works collaboratively with the agrochemical industry, to develop better formulations of existing insecticides and discovering and developing new insecticide molecules for the public health market.

Diagnostics

The number of skilled field entomologists able to accurately monitor and evaluate changes in insect vector populations has declined substantially over the last 40 years. The availability of trained staff and the lack of funding to employ such staff within the National Malaria Control Programmes (NMCPs) of Disease Endemic Countries mean that we need to re-align the old labour intensive entomological methods, using modern technology to develop cheap effective high throughput systems that are less labour intensive. These diagnostics also need to be able to rapidly feed information back into the NMCPs in a format that facilitates decision making. The IVCC is developing high throughput DNA-based diagnostics that can be used on dead mosquito collections, passively collected in fixed window traps by householders, to monitor mosquito population densities, their species, insecticide resistance status and malaria sporozoite infection rates (see Figure 1).

Development of these simple diagnostics has been massively facilitated by the availability of the *Anopheles gambiae* genome sequence. The programme has required painstaking use of state of the art molecular techniques, genomics, SNP mapping, QTL and Association mapping coupled to metabolism studies to identify the genes responsible for the insecticide resistance phenotype in the mosquitoes. Linking these resistance genes to SNP markers means that they can then be tracked using simple PCR reactions in the field. SNP markers for infection status, species identification and most of the pyrethroid resistance genes are now available for the major African malaria vector *Anopheles gambiae* [2-4], and a programme to develop similar markers is underway for *An. funestus* [5-7].

In the same resource poor settings there are also several requirements to monitor the efficacy, effectiveness and longevity of insecticide residues either on bednets or on wall treatments. Undertaking this by HPLC or other laboratory based methodologies is often beyond the resources of the Disease Endemic

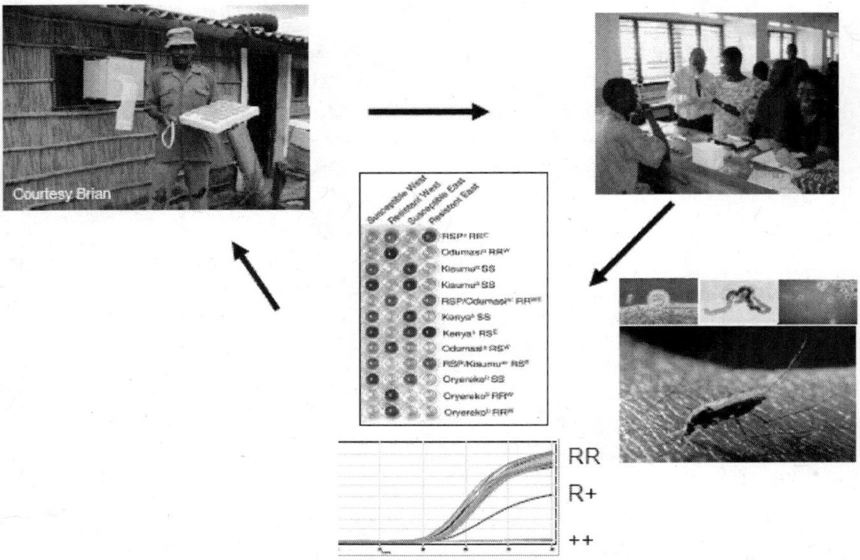

Figure 1. The collection and analysis of mosquito samples for insecticide resistance, infection status and species using passive collection methods and DNA based diagnostics.

Countries. The IVCC has therefore developed simple colorimetric based diagnostics assays that can be used rapidly, cheaply and safely in the field to establish whether treatments contain the biologically relevant level of insecticide to provide protection.

Software Systems

Although insecticide-based control of adult mosquitoes within the home has been central to malaria and dengue control for over 50 years, current tools to monitor the effectiveness of these interventions are poor. The IVCC, building on the pioneering work on malaria control monitoring and evaluation in southern Africa started by the late Dr Brian Sharp in Durban, South Africa[8,9], has developed operational scale software systems for monitoring the impact of interventions. The modular relational database system can be used by programmes to bring together a diversity of disease, operational treatment, entomological, spatial and geographical information to aid decisions on which interventions to implement and monitor their effectiveness once initiated. A similar dengue decision support system that can be implemented by municipalities responsible for responding to dengue outbreaks should revolutionise our ability to detect and appropriately respond to this rapidly spreading insect borne disease.

The malaria and dengue decision support systems, built of the same basic platform and operable in web and stand alone computer formats, will also allow us to rapidly assess new pesticide-based interventions, at scale, not only for their ability to kill insect and reduce insect population numbers, but also to define the impact of these new interventions, alone or in combination, on disease transmission.

While the underlying databases handling this information are complex (see Figure 2) the user interface is designed for deployment in disease endemic countries with data been easily downloaded and user interface screens largely driven by simple drop down menus. These systems are currently being evaluated at operational scale for malaria in southern Africa and by local municipalities for dengue in Mexico.

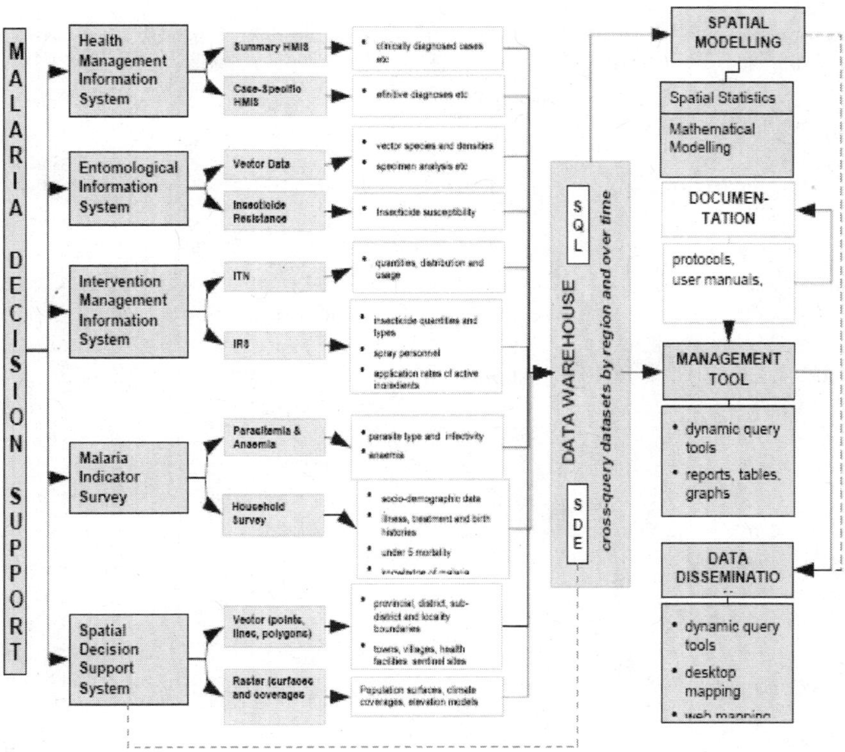

Figure 2. The modular database structure for collection of data needed for effective monitoring and evaluation of malaria control programmes.

New Public Health Pesticides and Formulations

Working with industry the IVCC aims to transform the vector control public health pesticide intervention landscape. To date there are only two well validated vector control systems that impact on disease transmission, the use of Long Lasting Insecticide Treated bednets (LLINs) and indoor residual spraying of insecticide (IRS). Larvicides in some urban settings may be cost effective but this intervention is not practical for deployment in rural settings where much of the disease transmission occurs.

DDT has been maintained for malaria control as, to date, it is the only insecticide IRS formulation that provides protection on all indoor surfaces for an entire transmission season (>6months) in hyperendemic countries after a single treatment. The IVCC has stimulated the development of new formulations of pyrethroids and organophosphates that should extend the lifespan of these treatments. We hope to see the launch of the first of these new products by the end of 2010.

Development of new active ingredients is a much longer and more expensive process. Projects entering the IVCC pipeline are taking one of two approaches; Molecular design against known insecticide target sites within the insect or high throughput screening of chemical libraries. A range of initial lead compounds will be defined over the next 18 months from these initial activities, which can then be refined. The goal is to develop three new insecticides with different modes of action over the next decade.

Consumer Products

Neither LLINs or IRS are ideal, both are costly to implement and neither are well received by many disease endemic country populations. The IVCC aims both to dramatically improve these interventions and to stimulate industry to bring new interventions to the market. We know that there is a large consumer market for coils, aerosols and insecticide impregnated mats, although these interventions in their current format are not cost effective and have no proven impact on disease transmission, being deployed by the consumers largely to reduce mosquito biting nuisance. Acting as in interface between the consumers, pesticide industry and other industrial and academic players the IVCC is already stimulating the development of novel insecticide-based interventions within the home and testing the efficacy of these interventions in reducing disease transmission.

Conclusions

Public Health Pesticides are an essential element of insect vector borne disease control programmes. PDPs have a major role in ensuring the stability of public health pesticide supply, engaging with industry to share the risk and plug expertise gaps to ensure that a robust pipeline of new insecticides is developed to replace older chemistries. New diagnostics that allow control programmes to monitor the effectiveness of their pesticide based interventions, and ensure that they are able to rapidly detect and respond to adverse changes in the insect vector population that are likely to result in increased disease transmission should ensure that the increased levels of international funds available for malaria and other vector borne disease control are used efficiently and effectively.

References

1. Hemingway J, Beaty BJ, Rowland M, Scott TW, Sharp BL. The Innovative Vector Control Consortium: improved control of mosquito-borne diseases. *Trends in Parasitology* 2006;**22**(7)**:**308-312.
2. Cohuet A, Krishnakumar S, Simard F, et al. SNP discovery and molecular evolution in *Anopheles gambiae,* with special emphasis on innate immune system. *BMC Genomics* 2008;**19**(9)**:**227.
3. Bass C, Williamson MS, Wilding C, Donnelly MJ, Field LM. Identification of the main malaria vectors in the Anopheles gambiae species complex using a TaqMan real-time PCR assay. *Malar J.* 2007;**6:**155.
4. Kulkarni MA, Rowland M, Alifrangis M, et al. Occurrence of the leucine-to-phenylalanine knockdown resistance (kdr) mutation in *Anopheles arabiensis* populations in Tanzania, detected by a simplified high-throughput SSOP-ELISA method. *Malar J.* 2006;**5**(56).
5. Wondji CS, Hemingway J, Ranson H. Identification and analysis of single nucleotide polymorphisms (SNPs) in the mosquito *Anopheles funestus,* malaria vector. *BMC Genomics* 2007;**8:**5.
6. Wondji CS, Hunt RH, Pignatelli P, et al. An integrated genetic and physical map for the malaria vector *Anopheles funestus*. *Genetics* 2005;**171**(4)**:**1779-87.
7. Wondji CS, Morgan J, Coetzee M, et al. Mapping a Quantitative Trait Locus (QTL) conferring pyrethroid resistance in the African malaria vector *Anopheles funestus*. *BMC Genomics* 2007;**8:**34.
8. Feachem R, Sabot O. A new global malaria eradication strategy. *The Lancet* 2008;**371**(9624)**:**1633-1635.
9. Kelly-Hope L, Ranson H, Hemingway J. Lessons from the past: managing insecticide resistance in malaria control and eradication programmes. *The Lancet Infectious Diseases* 2008;**8**(6)**:**387-389.

Current Status and Control Prices

Chapter 2

Pyrethroid resistance in the African mosquito *Anopheles gambiae* and alternative insecticides for indoor residual spraying and use on mosquito nets

Mark Rowland and Raphael N'Guessan

London School of Hygiene & Tropical Medicine, Keppel Street, London WC1E 7HT, UK

Resistance to pyrethroid insecticides has become widespread in *Anopheles gambiae* in West Africa. Whilst the kdr resistance in the *An. gambiae* S cytotype appears to have no operational importance, the resistance that has recently developed in the M cytotype of *An. gambiae* does appear to be protective and to threaten the future of pyrethroids at a time when coverage of insecticide treated nets and indoor residual spraying are being scaled up to great effect. There is an urgent need to develop alternative insecticides for vector control. No new class of chemistry has emerged for adult mosquito control since the pyrethroids. The primary characteristics required in an adulticide are contact activity, long residual activity and low mammalian toxicity. These criteria are less essential in agricultural insecticides where most R&D is focused. Two exceptions that may meet the vector control criteria are chlorfenapyr, a pyrrole, and indoxacarb, an oxadiazine used in crop protection. These compounds are unlikely to show cross-resistance to standard neurotoxic insecticides. Older chemistries such as the organophosphates have renewed potential in vector control. Advances in formulation technology mean that the residual activity of short lived insecticides may be extended to cover entire transmission seasons, reducing the need for costly, repeated applications. The problem of pyrethroid resistance in West Africa and the prospect of finding new compounds to supplement the pyrethroids are described. Such products will need to be evaluated in laboratory and field trials before they can be approved or taken up by malaria control programmes.

Insecticide treated nets (ITNs) are the most powerful malaria control tool to be developed since the advent of indoor residual spraying (IRS) in the 1940s (1). Twenty years after the trials which first demonstrated the potential impact of ITNs for reducing malaria morbidity and mortality, we are now witnessing the massive scale up of ITN coverage in Africa driven by national and international programs and supported among others by the Global Fund and President's Malaria Initiative. In some regions of countries the incidence of malaria has fallen considerably over the last few years and this is attributed in part to the increased coverage of ITNs and long-lasting insecticidal nets (LLIN) (2, 3). There is an air of optimism, and the recent call by the Bill & Melinda Gates Foundation to work towards the elimination or eradication of malaria is being taken seriously by international malaria control organizations and is stimulating new thinking and more ambitious targets.

What are the obstacles to achieving this ambitious goal? The financial requirements are huge and the commitment needs to be open ended. It is estimated that to provide 80% of children at risk with available malaria interventions will cost $1900 million per year (4). Each LLIN will have to be replaced every 3-5 years. Over time there will be competing demands for resources and changing health priorities. But if the present trends continue, and further inroads are made into malaria in subsaharan Africa or even elimination in fringe areas, there is reason to hope that political commitment and financial resources will continue. If there are checks on progress or reversals of trends the commitment might falter. What then are the potential technical or operational obstacles to success? In the long term, insecticide resistance is probably the most important threat. Chemical control success comes at a price, and the cost of controlling insect vectors is resistance. Over the last decade there has been one setback and one false alarm. In South Africa the pyrethroid resistance that evolved in *An. funestus* (an oxidase based detoxification mechanism) led to the failure of indoor residual spraying and to an epidemic of malaria (5). Only by switching to DDT and to carbamates was the problem overcome. The development of the site insensitivity pyrethroid resistance mechanism known as *kdr* in *An. gambiae* and its spread across West Africa have led to considerable alarm. With IRS there are alternatives to pyrethroids one can turn to. Not so with ITNs because only the pyrethroids are approved for this purpose (6). The selection of *kdr* is largely attributed to contamination of breeding sites by agricultural insecticides (7). Only after a series of field trials in experimental huts and a full scale malaria control trial of ITNs in a group of villages in Cote d'Ivoire was it concluded that this form of resistance poses no threat to the epidemiological effectiveness of ITNs (8, 9). But as we shall see, the situation it not quite so simple or clear cut as initially thought.

Alternative insecticides to pyrethroids that have potential for use on nets do exist. These originate from the agricultural sector. Most do not have the ideal set of attributes required of mosquito control agents such as low mammalian toxicity and long residual activity. Until recently there has been no great need to search for alternatives. But the situation is changing. A form of pyrethroid resistance has developed in An gambiae in West Africa that appears to have major operational significance and seems to be spreading fast (10, 11). The resistance needs to be investigated thoroughly and quickly so we can find ways to address it.

Potential alternative insecticides to the pyrethroids may be sought from older chemistries such as the organophosphates or carbamates (12, 8). These classes were superseded by the pyrethroids in the 1980s but may have renewed utility for vector control provided the former disadvantages such as short residual activity can be overcome through re-formulation. Other alternatives come from newer chemistries. Insecticides such as chlorfenapyr, a pyrrole, and indoxacarb, an oxadiazine were developed for crop and domestic pests and express both stomach and contact activity (10, 13). Chlorfenapyr has a novel mode of action, targeting the oxidative pathways in insect mitochondria. Indoxacarb acts on the sodium channels of the nervous system but at a different site to the pyrethroids. Both seem unlikely to show cross resistance to older classes of insecticide.

The development and evaluation of any new insecticide for vector control goes through three phases, reviewed recently by WHO (14). After initial testing for toxicity and activity on substrates in the laboratory, the insecticide goes forward for field testing in experimental huts as an IRS formulation or ITN treatment to investigate the toxic, residual and behavioural effects under more realistic conditions. The insecticide then goes forward to field testing in Phase III trials to determine the impact on mosquito populations and malaria transmission indicators. The techniques used in these 3 phases of evaluation are equally well suited for uncovering any negative impact of resistance on the continued effectiveness of ITNs or IRS.

In this paper we focus on trials undertaken in experimental huts in West and East Africa. We demonstrate the operational significance of resistance in W. African *An gambiae* and its impact on the efficacy of ITNs and IRS compared to an area of susceptibility. The second describes a series of evaluations of alternative insecticides as putative ITN or IRS control agents.

Materials and Methods

Study sites and mosquitoes

West Africa

Ladji is a village on the edge of Cotonou, capital of Benin. The *An. gambiae* is comprised of the Mopti (M) cytotype and shows resistance to pyrethroids and DDT with *kdr* present at 83% frequency and elevated oxidase and α-esterase activity than *An. gambiae* laboratory susceptible strains.

Malanville is in the north of Benin in an irrigated rice-growing valley. The local *An. gambiae* is comprised of the M cytotype but the *kdr* gene is almost absent and mosquitoes are susceptible to pyrethroids.

Yaokoffikro is the field site of the Institut Pierre Richet in Bouaké, Côte d'Ivoire, situated near rice and vegetable fields. The local *An. gambiae* is comprised of the S cytotype and the frequency of the *kdr* gene fluctuates around 90%. OP resistance due to $Ace\text{-}1^R$ is present at a frequency of 41%.

East Africa

Lower Moshi is an area of rice irrigation in Kilimanjaro region of Tanzania. The local vector is *An. arabiensis* and is susceptible.

Experimental huts

The style of experimental hut differs between W and E Africa. Huts are representative of house structures in the regions (15, 16). Both types are made from bricks with corrugated iron roofs. Ceilings are lined with hessian sackcloth on the interior surfaces. Walls are plastered with cement in the West and with mud in the East African design. Each hut is built on a concrete base surrounded by water-filled moat to exclude ants. Mosquito access is via window or eave slits. Verandah traps project from the wall of each hut. There are 6 huts at each site.

Mosquito net treatments

The nets were made of white 100-denier polyester netting. To simulate badly torn nets, 80 holes, each measuring 2cm x 2cm, were cut in the sides and ends of each net.

The pyrethroids used were formulations of lambdacyhalothrin (Syngenta, Switzerland): Icon 2.5% CS a microencapsulated suspension designed for ITN, Icon 10% WP a wettable powder designed for IRS.

The OP used was chlorpyrifos methyl 38.8% CS (Dow Agro Science, UK), an experimental microencapsulated suspension. The chlorfenapyr formulation was Phantom 15% SC (BASF Corp, USA). The indoxacarb formulation was Steward 15% SC (Dupont, USA).

The application rates were:

- lambdacyhalothrin 18mg/m^2 for ITN and 30mg/m^2 for IRS.
- chlorpyrifos methyl 100mg/m^2 for ITN and 500mg/m^2 for IRS.
- chlorfenapyr 100mg/m^2 for ITN.

Indoor residual treatments were applied using a hand-operated compression sprayer equipped with a flat fan nozzle. The control hut was sprayed with water only. Netting was treated by dipping in aqueous solution of the formulations.

Sleepers and mosquito collections

The treatments were randomly allocated to the experimental huts at each site. Volunteers slept overnight in the huts from 20:00 to 05:00 hours. Informed consent was given to participate in the study and chemoprophylaxis was provided. Ethical approval was granted by the LSHTM and Benin national ethics committees. The sleepers were rotated between huts to correct for possible variation in individual attractiveness. Each morning mosquitoes were collected from the floors, walls, and ceilings of rooms, verandahs and nets using aspirators and torches. Live mosquitoes were held for up to 72h and supplied with 10% honey solution before delayed mortality was scored.

The impact of each treatment was expressed relative to the control in terms of:

- Deterrence: the proportional reduction in the number of mosquitoes entering a treated hut relative to that entering the control hut.
- Blood-feeding inhibition: the reduction in blood feeding rate relative to the control hut.
- Mortality: the proportions of mosquitoes found dead in the hut up to 72h holding period.

The Benin trials of lambdacyhothrin ITN and IRS were undertaken in pyrethroid resistance (Ladji) and susceptible (Mellanville) areas. In Ivory Coast only lambdacyhothrin ITN was evaluated. Chlorpyrifos methyl was evaluated in Benin and Ivory Coast at the same time as lambdacyhalothrin. In the East African trial chlorfenapyr was evaluated only as an ITN treatment.

Residual activity of insecticide treatments

To evaluate residual activity WHO cone bioassays were undertaken each month using a laboratory susceptible strain of *An. gambiae* (Kisumu). Females, 3-5 days old, were exposed to nets for 3 min or to sprayed walls for 30 min and mortality recorded after 24h.

Laboratory bioassays

Laboratory evaluation of indoxacarb was limited to testing a range of dosages on netting in WHO cones against pyrethroid susceptible and resistant (*kdr*) strains of *An. gambiae*. The laboratory evaluation of chlorfenapyr against these two strains was made using a tunnel test with netting partition between the release chamber and the baited chamber (14).

Results

Lambdacyhalothrin ITNs and IRS

Benin trial

In Benin 1395 female *An. gambiae* M cytotype were collected in the hut trials at Ladji and 1523 in trials at Malanville. Fewer *An. gambiae* entered the ITN and IRS treated huts than the respective control huts. Resistance or susceptibility status made no difference to the proportion deterred (Table 1).

Table I. Summary of results of experimental hut trials of lambdacyhalothrin (LC) and chlorpyrifos-methyl (CM) treated nets (ITN) and indoor residual spraying (IRS) against *An. gambiae* in Benin and Ivory Coast. Ladji is an area with pyrethroid resistant M form *An. gambiae*, Melanville an area with pyrethroid susceptible S form and Yaokoffikro an area with pyrethroid resistant S form *An. gambiae*.

	ITN			IRS		
	Females[1]	% BF[2]	% M[3]	Females[1]	% BF[2]	% M[3]
Ladji						
Untreated	17.2[a]	82.0[a]	13.6[a]	5.1[a]	87.7[a]	12.3[a]
LC	9.7[b]	82.1[a]	29.8[b]	2.9[b]	73.5[a]	30.8[b]
CM	16.2[a]	78.9[a]	45.2[c]	10.5	82.0[a]	95.5[c]
Melanville						
Untreated	9.1[a]	77.7[a]	3.6[a]	12.5[a]	94.0[a]	1.4[a]
LC	6.7[b]	3.0[b]	98.5[b]	9.9[b]	69.6[b]	72.1[b]
CM						
Yaokoffikro						
Untreated	2.5[a]	38.6[a]	10.8[a]			
LC	1.0[b]	0[b]	67.6[b]			
CM	1.5[b]	6.0[c]	62.0[b]			

[1] Females = females caught per night.
[2] % BF = % blood-fed.
[3] % M = % mortality.

The untreated net was no obstacle to blood-feeding of *An. gambiae* at either Ladji or Melanville owing to the large number of holes. Treatment of the holed nets with pyrethroid led to a 96% reduction in the number of mosquitoes blood-feeding at the insecticide susceptible site (Malanville) but to no reduction in blood-feeding at the resistance site (Ladji) (Table 1).

At Malanville, both modes of treatment were highly insecticidal, the ITN killing 99% and the IRS killing 72% of *An. gambiae* that entered the huts.

At Ladji, the proportions killed in the ITN and IRS treated huts were never greater than 30% (Table 1).

Relative to the control huts, lambdacyhalothrin treated nets and IRS induced little or no exiting of the pyrethroid resistant mosquitoes into the verandahs of the Ladji huts, despite high survival rate of mosquitoes in the huts. At Malanville, pyrethroid induced repellency by ITN or IRS was not evident, and may have been obscured by the high mortality rates in the room of the hut.

Ivory Coast trial

In Ivory Coast 59% where the *An. gambiae* S cytotype is prevalent fewer females entered the hut with lamdacyhalothrin ITN than entered the hut with the untreated net.

A smaller proportion of *An. gambiae* females fed through the untreated net in the Ivory Coast than in the Benin trials (Table 1). None of the *kdr* resistant mosquitoes managed to feed through the holed ITN, in marked contrast to the situation in S. Benin. The mortality rates in the ITN hut was 67.6%. Compared to the resistance in Benin the resistance in Ivory Coast seemed to provide no obstacle to the continuing effectiveness of ITNs.

Chlorpyrifos methyl treated ITNs and IRS

Benin trial

In Benin the number of mosquitoes entering the huts with chlorpyrifos methyl treated ITN or IRS did not differ from the respective untreated controls – hence there was no evidence of deterrence or spatial repellency with this OP (Table 1).

In Benin blood-feeding rates in huts with chlorpyrifos methyl treated ITN or IRS were no different from the untreated control or lambdacyhalothrin huts – hence there was no evidence of contact irritancy or feeding inhibition with chlorpyrifos methyl (Table 1). In contrast, in Ivory Coast, with *An gambiae* S form, blood-feeding rates were lower in the chlorpyrifos methyl huts than in the control huts but not as low as in the lamdacyhalothrin hut (Table 1).

In Benin mortality rates with the chlorpyrifos methyl treated ITN were significantly higher than with the pyrethroid treated ITN. Mortality rates with the chlorpyrifos methyl IRS treatment was exceptionally high (95%) against this pyrethroid resistant population compared to lambdacyhalothrin. Cone bioassays of the chlorpyrifos methyl treated cement walls showed no loss of activity during the 11 month follow up period (Figure 1). Hence chlorpyrifos methyl has the attributes of toxicity and longevity required to control pyrethroid resistant populations of *An. gambiae.*

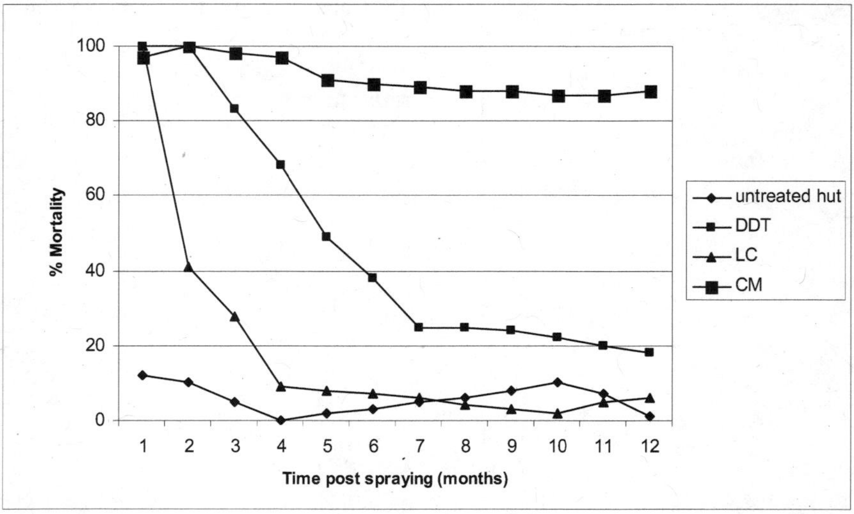

Figure 1. Residual activity of sprayed insecticide on cement walls of experimental huts as determined in WHO cone bioassay tests. LC = lambdacyhalothrin WP, CM = chlorpyrifos methyl CS.

Ivory Coast trial

In Ivory Coast mortality with the chlorpyrifos methyl ITN was 62%, a similar level of mortality to that in Benin, despite the presence of OP resistance due to insensitive acetylcholinesterase *Ace-1*^{R} (Table 1).

Chlorfenapyr treated ITNs and IRS

Tanzanian trial

The number of mosquitoes entering the huts with chlorfenapyr and deltamethrin treated ITNs did not differ from the number entering the control hut – hence there was no evidence of deterrence or spatial repellency with this pyrrole insecticide (Table 2).

Blood feeding rates in huts with chlorfenapyr ITN were 36.6% lower than in the untreated hut and similar to feeding rates in the huts with the deltamethrin ITN.

Mortality rates with the chlorfenapyr treated ITN was similar to that in huts with the pyrethroid treated ITN.

Table II. Summary of results obtained for *Anopheles arabiensis* in experimental huts comparing chlorfenapyr and deltamethrin. Numbers in the same row sharing a letter superscript do not differ significantly.

	Untreated Net	*Chlorfenapyr 100mg/m²*	*Deltamethrin 25mg/m²*
Females caught/night (total)	26.8 (321)	35.2 (422)	19.8 (238)
Blood feeding %	39.6[a]	25.1[b]	22.3[b]
Blood feeding inhibition %	-	36.6	43.7
Mortality %	4.7a	56.9[b]	49.6[b]
Immediate mortality[1]	0.0[a]	30.4[b]	34.7[b]
Exiting rates %	81.9[a]	81.0[a]	88.2[a]
% caught in net	10.9[a]	7.8[ab]	3.8[b]

[1] % of total mortality.

Benin trial

The number of mosquitoes entering the huts with chlorfenapyr treated ITN and IRS did not differ from the control huts – once again there was no evidence of spatial repellency (Table 3).

Blood feeding rates in huts with chlorfenapyr IRS were 17% lower than in the untreated hut. Feeding rates in huts with the treated ITN were no different from in huts with untreated nets.

Mortality rates with the chlorfenapyr treated ITN and IRS (Table 3) were significantly higher than with the pyrethroid treated ITN or IRS in the earlier trial (Table 1). Hence chlorfenapyr shows potential for overcoming pyrethroid resistant mosquitoes. Residual activity was not sustained on either ITNs or IRS for more than 6 weeks. The formulation was never designed for long residual activity on these types of substrate.

Table III: Summary results of experimental hut trial of chlorfenapyr treated nets (ITN) and indoor residual spraying (IRS) against *An. gambiae* M form (pyrethroid-resistant) at the Ladji field station.

	ITN		IRS	
	Untreated net	Treated[1]	Untreated hut	Treated[1]
Total	84	116	199	310
% exiting	32.1	31.9	52.3	48.1
% bloodfed	91.7	87.1	52.3	48.1
% blood feeding inhibition	-	5.0	-	17.7
% dead	9.5	53.5	8.5	82.9

[1] Chlorfenapyr 1 g/m^2.

Resistance tests

In laboratory tunnel tests the trend in mortality was similar between susceptible and pyrethroid resistant strains of *An. gambiae* and hence there was no evidence of cross resistance between pyrethroids and chlorfenapyr (Figure 2).

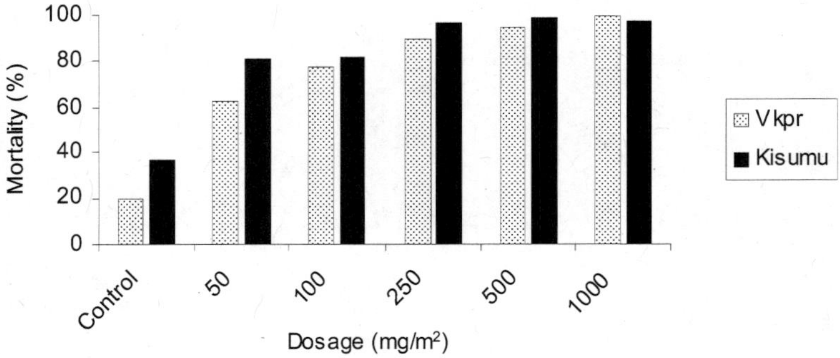

Figure 2. Results of tunnel tests with chlorfenapyr treated netting against pyrethroid resistant (Vkpr) and susceptible (Kisumu) strains of *An. gambiae*

Indoxacarb treated ITNs

Cone bioassays with indoxacarb treated netting showed a typical dosage-mortality response against the susceptible Kisumu and pyrethroid resistant Vkpr strains and hence no evidence of cross resistance (Figure 3). The insecticide was slow acting, taking up to 72h to kill.

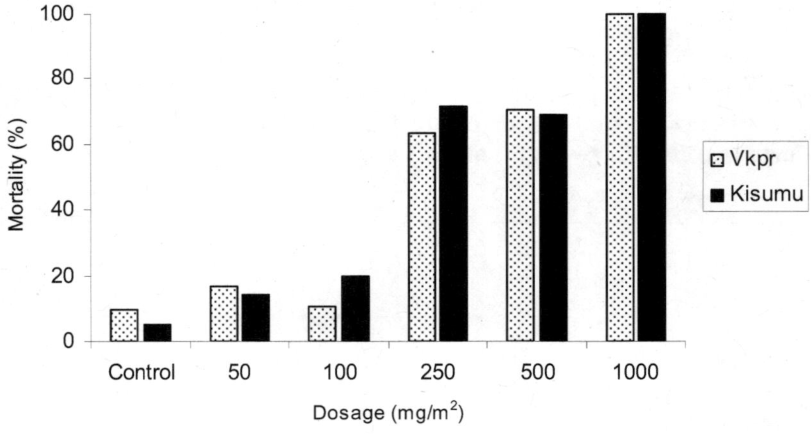

Figure 3. Results of WHO cone tests with indoxacarb treated netting against pyrethroid resistant (Vkpr) and susceptible (Kisumu) strains of *An. gambiae*

Discussion

There was a major loss of pyrethroid efficacy associated with resistance in *An. gambiae* at Ladji, southern Benin. The reduction in efficacy affected IRS and ITNs equally, and it is unlikely that the small proportion of insects that were killed by the insecticide would lead to any reduction in transmission.

Once holed the ITNs were no barrier to resistant mosquitoes which then went on to blood-feed on the occupants. There was a degree of personal protection associated with pyrethroid ITNs and IRS as fewer mosquitoes entered these huts. Whether this would hold true for houses with multiple routes of entry is unknown.

The hut results from southern Benin contrast with the results from an area of Ivory Coast which had a comparable frequency of *kdr* to that of Ladji but where lambdacyhalothrin treated ITN induced much higher mortality rates. The differences in the results are associated with differences in the species type, the Ivorian *An. gambiae* being the S molecular form whereas the Beninoise *An. gambiae* is the M form. M and S types differ in ecological distribution and habitat and also it would seem in their behaviour and ability to withstand contact or penetrate holed ITNs. The M type may express elevated levels of multi-function oxidases (17) suggesting the possibility that *kdr* and elevates MFOs together provide a level of resistance that renders ITNs and IRS ineffective.

The present study provides strong evidence that pyrethroid resistance in Benin is capable of undermining control measures based on ITN and IRS. Evidence is emerging that the problem is extending beyond the frontiers of Benin. During recent hut trials in Burkina Faso it was realised that the M form had become predominant over the space of a year making the ITNs under test relatively ineffective (18). On the island of Bioko on the West African coast, IRS campaigns with pyrethroid failed to curtail an increase in the population of *An. gambiae* M form, and there was further selection of *kdr* during the spraying campaign. It required switching to the carbamate bendiocarb before the mosquito population, and malaria, went into decline (11).

Further work to measure the epidemiological impact of resistance is urgently needed. This can be done in village randomised trials of ITNs and IRS, ideally in two areas, one with a high frequency and one with a low frequency of resistance.

The need to develop alternative insecticides to replace or supplement pyrethroids on nets or IRS is becoming urgent, and should be put on a par with the seeking of new antimalarial drugs or vaccines that have received far greater attention and resources in recent years. Developing a long lasting organophosphate IRS formulation is, as the results show, feasible. The prospect of finding alternative compounds for use on nets is more daunting. Compared to other classes of insecticide, pyrethroids are extremely safe for people, do very little damage to the environment, and are highly toxic to insects. Their rapid mode of action and excito-repellent effects are especially important for personal protection. There are other insecticides that might be as effective in small quantities as pyrethroids, but some of these (e.g. the carbamates) may not be safe enough for use on nets (19). Other alternatives, described here, are safe but are relatively non repellent, so might be good at killing blood-seeking mosquitoes and transmission control but less good at preventing mosquitoes from biting the occupant of the net. Use of a non-repellent or slow acting insecticide alternative in combination with a pyrethroid may provide a toxic and repellent cocktail and may reduce the rate of selection of pyrethoid resistance (20, 8). The exploring of alternative insecticides has not received the attention it deserves, but is now a more active area of research, and it is likely that one or more non-pyrethroid compounds will prove to be suitable for use on nets in the future. Unless a pipeline of products suitable for use on nets is quickly developed the strategy to scale up ITN use will be compromised and the present gains in malaria control will not be sustained.

References

1. Hill, J.; Lines, J.; Rowland, M. *Advances in Parasitology* **2006,** *61*, 77-128.
2. Okiro, A. E.; Hay, S. I.; Gikandi, P. W.; Sharif, S. K.; Noor, A. M.; Peshu, N.; Marsh, K.; Snow, R. W. *Malaria Journal* **2007**, *6*, 151.
3. Bhattarai, A.; Ali, S. A.; Kachur, P. S.; Martensson, A.; Abbas, A. K.; Khatib, R., Al-mafazy, A.; Ramsan, M.; Rotllant, G.; Gerstenmaier, J. F.; Molteni, F.; Abdulla, S.; Montgomery, S. M.; Kaneko, A.; Bjorkman, A. *PLoS Medicine* **2007**, *4*.
4. WHO, 2005. 58th World Health Assembly: Malaria report by the Secretariat. WHO58.8.
5. Hargreaves. K.; Koekemoer, L. L.; Brooke, B. D.; Hunt, R. H.; Mthembu, J.; Coetzee, M. *Medical and Veterinary Entomology* **2000**, *14*, 181-189.
6. Zaim, M.; Guillet, P. *Trends in Parasitology* **2002**, *18*, 161-163.
7. Chandre, F.; Darriet, F.; Duchon, S.; Finot, L.; Manguin, S.; Carnevale, P.; Guillet, P. *Medical and Veterinary Entomology* **2000**, *14*, 81-88.
8. Asidi, A. N.; N'Guessan, R.; Koffi, A. A.; Curtis, C. F.; Hougard, J. M.; Chandre, F.; Corbel, V.; Darriet, F.; Zaim, M.; Rowland, M. W. *Malaria Journal* **2005**, *4*, 25.
9. Henry, M. C.; Assi, S. B.; Rogier, C.; Dossou–Yovo, J.; Chandre, F.; Guillet, P.; Carnevale, P. *American Journal of Tropical Medicine and Hygiene* **2005**, *73*, 859–64.
10. N'Guessan, R.; Corbel, V.; Bonnet, J.; Yates, A.; Asidi, A.; Boko, P.; Odjo, A.; Akogbeto, M.; Rowland, M. *Journal of Medical Entomology* **2007,** *44,* 270-276.
11. Sharp, B. L.; Ridl, F. C.; Govender, D.; Kuklinski, J.; Kleinschmidt, I. *Malaria Journal* **2007**, *6*, 52.
12. Kolaczinski, J. H.; Fanello, C.; Herve, J. P.; Conway, D. J.; Carnevale, P.; Curtis, C. F. *Bulletin of Entomological Research* **2000**, *90*, 125-132.
13. N'Guessan, R.; Corbel, V.; Akogbéto, M.; Rowland, M. *Emerging Infectious Diseases* **2007**, *13*, 199-206.
14. WHO, 2006. Guidelines for testing mosquito adulticides for indoor residual spraying and treatment of mosquito nets. WHO/CDS/NTD/WHOPES/GCDPP/2006.3

15. Asidi, A. N.; N'Guessan, R.; Hutchinson, R. A.; Traore–Lamizana, M.; Carnevale, P.; Curtis, C. F. *Medical and Veterinary Entomology* **2004**, *18*, 134–40.
16. Mosha, F. W.; Lyimo, I. N. Oxborough, R. M.; Matowo, J.; Malima, R.; Feston, E.; Mndeme, R.; Tenu, F.; Kulkarni, M.; Maxwell, C. A.; Magesa, S. M.; Rowland, M. W. *Annals of Tropical Medicine and Parasitology* **2008**, *102*, 367–376.
17. Corbel, V.; N'Guessan, R.; Brengues, C.; Chandre, F.; Djogbenou, L.; Martin, T.; Akogbéto, M.; Hougard, J. M.; Rowland, M. *Acta Tropica* **2007**, *101*, 207-216.
18. WHO, 2008. Report of the eleventh WHOPES working group meeting, WHO/HQ, Geneva. 10–13 December 2007, Review of: Spinosad 7.48% DT, Netprotect®, Duranet®, Dawaplus®, ICON® Maxx
19. Guillet, P.; N'Guessan, R.; Darriet, F.; Traore–Lamizana, M. *Medical and Veterinary Entomology* **2001,** *15*, 105-112.
20. Hougard, J. M.; Corbel, V.; N'Guessan, R.; Darriet, F.; Chandre, F.; Akogbeto, M.; Baldet, T.; Guillet, P.; Carnevale, P.; Traore-Lamizana, M. *Bulletin of Entomological Research* **2003**, *93*, 491-198.

Chapter 3

Insecticide Resistance in the Mosquito *Culex pipiens* Complex

Concerns about development of pyrethroid resistance

Osamu Komagata, Shinji Kasai and Takashi Tomita

Department of Medical Entomology, National Institute of Infectious Diseases,
1-23-1 Toyama, Shinjuku-ku, Tokyo 162-8640, Japan

We investigated insecticide susceptibility of the mosquito *Culex pipiens* complex in Japan, using a total of 56 field-collected colonies of *Cx. pipiens molestus*, *Cx. p. pallens*, and *Cx. quinquefasciatus*. In 4 larvicides bioassayed (fenitrothion, etofenprox, diflubenzuron, and pyriproxyfen), obviously reduced susceptibilities were observed for a pyrethroid etofenprox. Twenty-two colonies exhibited over 10% survival rates at 5.7 μg/ml etofenprox concentration, which is 10 times higher than the practical concentration. Etofenprox resistant strains of *Cx. p. m.* and *Cx. p. pallens* were established by larval selections in the laboratory. The selected strains exhibited 10^3 order etofenprox resistance and also cross resistance to permethrin and phenothrin. The major mechanisms of pyrethroid resistance in these strains were both increased detoxifying activities of cytochrome P450 monooxygenases and *kdr* mutations in the sodium channel gene. *kdr* mutations identified from *Cx. p. m.* and *Cx. p.*

pallens were L1014F and L1014S, respectively. Microarray analysis was conducted, targetting larval gene expressions of 62 different cytochrome P450 isoforms, using pyrethroid resistant JPP strain and a susceptible strains of *Cx. q*. Two extraordinarily highly expressing P450 genes, CYP9M10 and CYP4H34, were identified in JPP. The larva-specific expressions of the two P450 genes in JPP mosquitoes conformed to a great decrease in permethrin-resistance in adults, suggesting these isoforms are likely involved in pyrethroid detoxification.

Introduction

Culex pipiens complex is the major vector mosquito of lymphatic Filariasis and West Nile fever. In Japan, three sibling species are distributed: *Culex pipiens pallens*, *Culex pipiens molestus*, and *Culex quinquefasciatus*. Generally, *Cx. p. pallens* and *Cx. p. m.* are distributed in the temperate and subarctic regions, whereas *Cx. quinquefasciatus* distributes in the tropical or subtropical regions. Morphologically, these 3 species are similar and fairly difficult to distinguish, but there are some physiological differences. *Cx. p. m.* usually inhabits underground areas or lives in enclosed dark spaces where blood sources are limited so that females lay the first egg raft without feeding on blood (autogeny). In addition, this species has the ability to copulate in a narrow space (stenogamy) and to breed without diapause (homodynamy). Because the primary habitat of *Cx. p. m.* is the underground area of buildings, a well known nuisance area in Japan, they tend to be the target of control by insecticides. Moreover, the development of resistance to organophosphates in *Cx. p. m.* was reported in Japan (1).

In the United States, the West Nile fever has been ongoing since 1999. The transmission cycle of West Nile virus is alternately rotated between birds and mosquitoes (2). An incidental bite from an infected mosquito causes infection of the virus in humans. Effective control of *Culex* mosquitoes is thus essential to prevent people from developing West Nile fever or West Nile encephalitis. The application of appropriate insecticides is one of the important means for controlling vector mosquitoes. However, continuous use of insecticide has resulted in the emergence worldwide of mosquitoes with developed resistance to various kinds of insecticides.

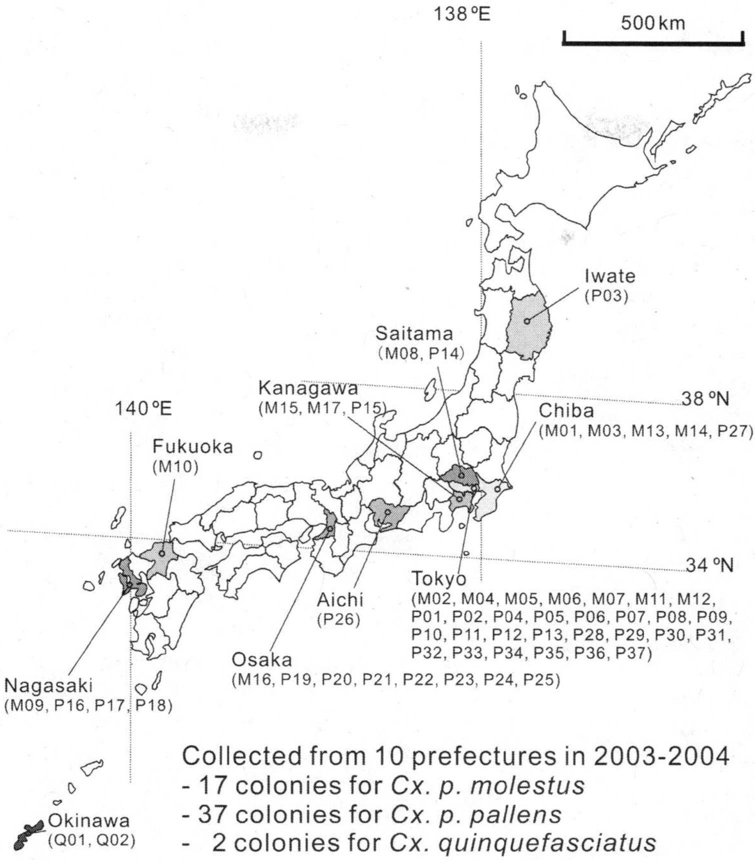

Figure 1. Localities of the field-collected colonies of *Cx. pipiens* complex. Code numbers for colonies correspond to those described in Figure 2.

To date, West Nile virus has not been confirmed in Japan, but if it lands in this country, the control of mosquitoes by insecticides will be the primary solution to the epidemic of the disease. In such a case, it will be crucial to know the status of the insecticide susceptibilities of the vector mosquitoes to be able to develop the best control strategy to prevent or minimize resistant development. Thus, it is necessary to conduct broad geographical surveys of mosquito susceptibilities to insecticides in advance of any such outbreak and to calculate the likely effectiveness of insecticide for use in an emergency. However, insecticide susceptibility of mosquitoes has recently only been rarely examined in Japan, where the incidence of Japanese encephalitis has decreased, and other mosquito-borne diseases such as filariasis and dengue have not been prevalent for the past 40 yr (3, 4). Herein, we report the current status of insecticide susceptibilities of *Cx. pipiens* complex to four insecticides, with four different modes of action, including organophosphate, pyrethroid, and insect growth regulator (IGR). Possible mechanisms of the resistance were also investigated.

Insecticide susceptibilities of field-collected mosquitoes

We collected mosquito samples across Japan and examined the susceptibilities of *Cx. p. m.* (17 colonies), *Cx. p. pallens* (37 colonies), and *Cx. q.* (2 colonies) (Figure 1) in 2003 and 2004 and then tested these colonies for larval susceptibility to representative larvicides. Before the study, we conducted bioassays for four insecticides (fenitrothion, etofenprox, diflubenzuron, and pyriproxyfen) using a standard susceptible strain of *Cx. p. pallens* (Horaana), and we estimated the LC_{99} values for each insecticide (5). Then, we configured three diagnostic concentrations (LC_{99} X1, X10, and X100) for the susceptible strain.

Fenitrothion is one of the most popular mosquitocides in Japan so that decreased sensitivity to this insecticide compared with the other insecticides was expected. However, against expectation, fenitrothion exhibited high efficacy against the *Culex* larvae (Figure 2). The working concentration of fenitrothion recommended by the manufacturer (the dosage regimen) is 2.0 μg/ml, but we detected a 0% survival rate even at 0.33 μg/ml (LC_{99} X10), showing that fenitrothion is still effective at present.

Twenty-two colonies showed survival rate of 10% at the diagnostic concentration of LC_{99} X100 of etofenprox (Figure 2). Because the total number of colonies was 56, overall 37% of the colonies contained resistant larvae, which survived at 5.7 μg/ml etofenprox. It is noteworthy that 3 colonies (Chiba, Yokohama, and Fukuoka, as shown by M13, M17, and M10 codes in the figure, respectively) of *Cx. p. molestus* exhibited a 100% survival rate at LC_{99} X100, suggesting that selection pressures by pyrethroid insecticides were extremely high in these environments.

The chitin synthesis inhibitor diflubenzuron was relatively effective against *Culex* larvae in Japan (Figure 2). We detected only one colony (Yokohama (M17)) exhibiting a relatively high level of resistance to diflubenzuron. The survival rate of the Yokohama colony was 47% at LC_{99} X100 (0.92 μg/ml). Because the working concentration of diflubenzuron is 0.5-1.25 μg/ml, our results exhibited that diflubenzuron is effective enough at present in Japan.

Another non-neuron target insecticide, pyriproxyfen, exhibited a slightly lower effectiveness as compared with diflubenzuron (Figure 2). However, the diagnostic concentration of pyriproxyfen was much lower than the working concentration of this insecticide so that pyriproxyfen is still sufficiently effective to control *Culex* larvae at present. The percentage of colonies that showed survival rates of 10% at LC_{99} X100 was zero (0/37) in *Cx. p. pallens* but 30% (5/17) in *Cx. p. m.*, which may reflect the recent intensive use of pyriproxyfen in the regular control activity taken against *Cx. p. m.* in Japan. Thus it is expected that additional selection induced by pyriproxyfen in the fields may result in the appearance of resistant colonies in the future.

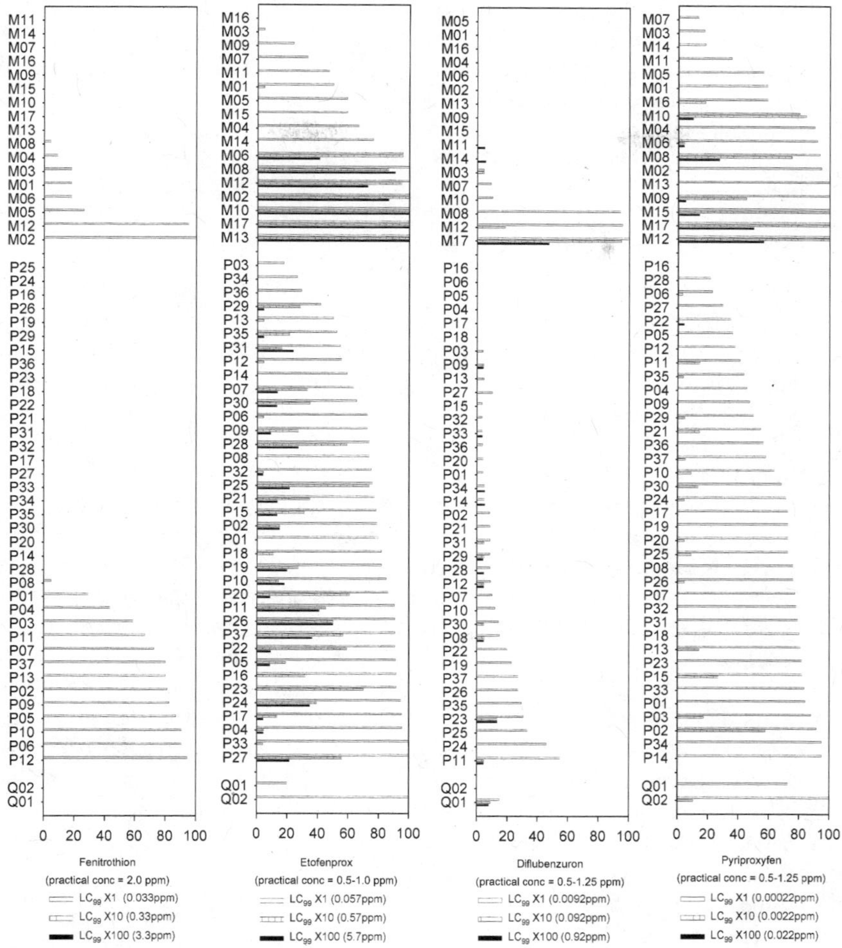

Figure 2. Survival rate of *Culex pipiens* complex collected from Japan exposed to 4 insecticides at 3 diagnostic concentrations which were calculated according to the toxicities against a susceptible strain (*LC*99 X1, X10, X100). See Figure 1 for the respective sampling areas.

Resistance level for etofenprox

The LC_{50} values to etofenprox were determined for *Cx. p. m.* colonies in which larval resistance levels were extremely high. The resistance ratios for Fukuoka (M10), Yokohama (M17), Chiba (M13), Shibuya (M02), Shinjuku (M06), and Otemachi (M12) as compared to the susceptible strain Horaana, were >2,307 (LC_{50} >60 ppm), 1,923 (>50 μg/ml), 1,050 (27.3 μg/ml), 919 (23.9 μg/ml), 527 (13.7 μg/ml), and 396 (10.3 μg/ml), respectively. The resistance ratios for etofenprox exceeded 300-fold in most colonies of *Cx. p. m.* and surprisingly, the LC_{50}s of two colonies exceeded 50 μg/ml, clearly suggesting that the selection pressure by pyrethroid was tremendously high in the field where these colonies were collected. Although we found that several colonies of *Cx. p. molestus* have developed high level of resistance to the active ingredient (etofenprox), the actual pesticide product sold on the market in Japan contains a synergist (S-421) so that our results do not necessarily mean that the etofenprox product are useless against mosquitoes in the field.

Cross resistance among pyrethroid compounds

By any measure, why did mosquitoes show resistance to etofenprox? This compound is relatively unpopular as a larvicide in Japan compared with fenitrothion or pyriproxyfen. To examine the resistance levels to other pyrethroids, we conducted bioassays with a resistant colony of *Cx. p. m.* (Fukuoka (M10)) for permethrin and phenothrin. The Fukuoka colony showed cross-resistance to permethrin and phenothrin, with the resistance ratios of 299- and 1,200-fold, respectively. These insecticides are popular as mosquito adulticides in Japan, so that it might be possible that the control of mosquitoes with these pyrethroids caused cross-resistance to etofenprox in larvae.

Several questions exist with regard to the etofenprox resistance of *Cx. p. pallens*. The major larval habitat of this mosquito species is aboveground open spaces, such as catch basins of parks or streets, and drains. In recent years in Japan, these areas tend to be less likely targeted for mosquito control, and active and mass control of mosquitoes is restricted to *Cx. p. m.* living under buildings. Then, why, how, and when did *Cx. p. pallens* develop resistance to the pyrethroids? One possible factor is that this mosquito species might had been selected by DDT which was used to control medically important pests in the post-World War II period. DDT was used in various applications to control mosquitoes as well as head and body lice. Because the target site of both pyrethroids and DDT is the sodium channel, the *kdr* (knockdown resistance) factor may have been selected by DDT several decades ago and remained up to the present. Moreover, Asahina reported that not only *Cx. p. m.* but also *Cx. p. pallens*, collected at a lumber yard in Tokyo in 1962, exhibited a high level of resistance to DDT (6). As another possibility, *Cx. p. pallens* could be selected by mosquito coils and their allied products. These products have been popular in Japan since 100 yr ago, and they are still widely used in most homes in the mosquito season. The active ingredients of these products are pyrethroids such as allethrin, pyrethrin, furamethrin, and so on. Therefore, selective pressure on the *Cx. p. pallens* population has been continuously sustained, even in recent Japan.

Decreased nerve sensitivity due to point mutations

Decreased sensitivity of the target site (sodium channel), the so called *kdr*-factor, is known to be a mechanism of pyrethroid resistance and insects that possess this feature display cross-resistance to multiple pyrethroids (7). We tested point mutations at a Leu in DIIS6 trans-membrane region (L1014, the position number follows *Musca domestica* orthologue) of *para*-orthologous sodium channel gene. At least 7 (M01, M02, M6, M10, M12, M13, and M17) of 17 *Cx. p. molestus* colonies segregated typical *kdr* genes (L1014F). At least 5 (P04, P06, P07, P11, and P37) of 37 *Cx. p. pallens* colonies segregated atypical *kdr* genes (L1014S). In order to investigate mosquito subspecies-specific segregation of the typical and atypical *kdr* genes, adult mosquitoes were collected in 2005 at two sites which are located in Shinjuku-ku, Tokyo. The two sites are apart by 2 km and thus the mosquitoes collected showed almost sympatric emergence. A total of 70 *Cx. p. molestus* and 15 *Cx. p. pallens* adults were individually tested for the *kdr* mutations. As a result, 29 *Cx. p. m.* and 3 *Cx. p. pallens* adults were carrying F1014 and S1014 genes, respectively, in heterozygous condition with the wild L1014 gene or homozygously (8). These results suggest that *Cx. p. m.* and *Cx. p. pallens* seldom hybridize in fields.

The S1014 mutation was originally found in a pyrethroid resistant strain of *Cx. p.* mosquitoes (Martinez-Torres et al. 1999). The significance of this mutation for pyrethroid resistance is supported from other study (Kasai, unpublished) as follows: the RNS strain originally segregating the Ser mutant allele less than 20% in Rinshi colony (P37) were subjected to larval selection with etofenprox for 7 generations and the allele finally come to homogeneous, suggesting that the Ser1014 mutation also confers pyrethroid resistance.

Increased detoxification due to P450 monooxygenase activity

In addition to *kdr*, detoxification enzymes also play very important roles in pyrethroid resistance. We tested the synergism of a general inhibitor of cytochrome P450 monooxygenases (abbr. P450s), piperonyl butoxide (PBO), with etophenprox, using 4th instar larvae from 8 strains of *Cx. p.* complex: JPal-per (abbr. JPP) strain of Cx. q. of Saudi Arabia origin and 7 strains which were derived from the field-collected domestic colonies above mentioned (M01, M06, M10, M12, M13, M17, and P37). The three of these strains derived from M06, M12, and P37 colonies were obtained after larval selection with etophenprox in laboratory and the otherwise denoted were directly derived from their original colonies without insecticidal selection. The JPP strain displays cross-resistance to several kinds of pyrethroids (9) and the major mechanism of this resistance has been demonstrated to be enhanced activities of P450s (10). The resistance ratio for JPP was 1,615 and those for the 7 domestic resistant strains ranged 879 to 2,282. The synergism ratio (i.e. [synergism effect to R strain] / [synergism effect to S strain] for JPP was 27 and those for the 7 domestic resistant strains ranged 9.4 to 179 (Kasai, unpublished). Therefore, increased detoxification due to P450 monooxygenase activity seems to tale over a major part in overall resistance.

Two notably overexpressing P450 genes in JPP larvae

We mostly originally isolated 62 different P450 cDNA sequences (16 known and 46 new sequences) of *Cx. pipiens* complex., based on degenerate PCR. The PCR primers were designed to target conserved insect P450 sequences. We then analyzed up- and down-regulations for the 62 P450 genes in JPP strain in contrast with an insecticide susceptible strain OGS of *Cx. q.* by oligonucleotide microarray experiments, using the obtained P450 cDNA sequences for microarray probes. The results involved 10 cases of two times or more up-regulation and 4 cases of one-half or less down-regulation in 62 cases of comparisons. The tentative code names or CYP names of up-regulated P450s (with the respective microarray ratios) were CYP4-like P1 (2.1-folds), CYP4D40 (2.6), CYP4H34 (9.4), CYP9M10 (50), CYP6-like P49 (2.2), CYP6-like P52 (2.8), CYP6Z1 (2.8), CYP6M12 (2.6), CYP6BB3 (2.3), and CYP6E1 (2.3). (Komagata, unpublished). The results suggest that not a small number of P450 isoforms may take part in the metabolism of pyrethroids in JPP mosquitoes.

Six P450 genes which exhibited over two-folds microarray ratios and also higher absolute transcription levels in JPP strain were picked up. Then the 6 genes were subjected to more accurate quantification, qPCR (Figure 3), where each P450 mRNA level is presented in contrast with a housekeeping gene, ribosomal protein subunit 3 (RPS3). CYP9M10 exhibited an absolutely high mRNA level, exceeding the level of RPS3. CTP6Z10 and then CYP4H34 genes subsequently followed the level of P32 gene in JPP. The transcription ratios for P32 and P14 in JPP (compared with the susceptible strain OGS) were expressed as 365- and 17.8-folds, respectively. The both absolutely high transcription level (in contrast with RPS3 gene expression in JPP strain) and extraordinarily high transcription ratios (JPP strain/OGS strain) for CYP9M10 and CYP4H34 were specific to JPP strain of *Cx. q.* and not demonstrated with the 5 etofenprox-resistant strains (derived from M01, M06, M10, M12, and M17 of *Cx. p. m.* and P37 of *Cx. p. pallens*) (Komagata, unpublished), even though both 10^3 level etofenprox resistance and a substantial contribution of elevated P450 activity were uniformly demonstrated with all these strains. Thus it is suggested that P450 isoforms other than CYP9M10 and CYP4H34 are also potentially involved in the resistance mechanisms. One such P450 might be CYP4Z10. Although its up-regulations in 5 resistant strains (JPP stain and the strains derived from M01, M06, M12, and M17, and P37 colonies) were moderate (around 2-folds) in contrast with the pairwised susceptible strains, the impact of elevated CYP4Z10 seems deep because its absolute transcription levels were uniformly as high as RPS3 gene.

Developmental changes in relative transcriptional levels for CYP9M10 and CYP4H34 were observed with JPP mosquitoes after standardized with RPS3 by

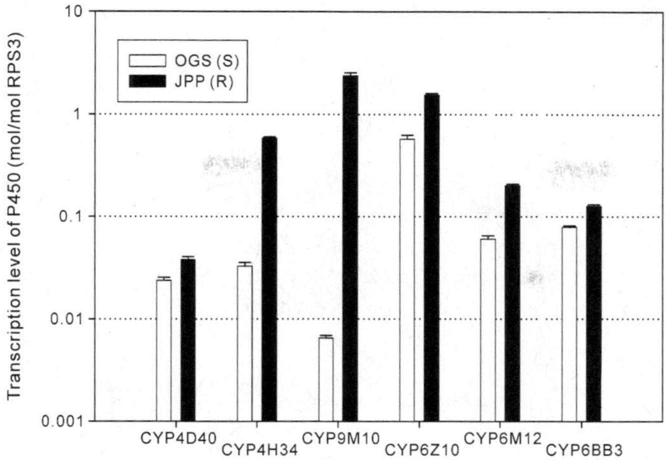

Figure 3. Relative transcription levels of 6 P450 genes measured by qPCR. The transcription level of each P450 gene in insecticide susceptible OGS and pyrethroid resistant JPP strains is standardized by molar amount of ribosomal protein subunit 3 (RPS3) transcript.

qPCR (not shown). The both genes had common features of an abundant larval expression especially in 4th instar larvae, and the traces of expression in embryos, pupae, and both male and female adults (Komagata, unpublished). Given that the extraordinary genetic overexpressions of the two genes are conferring (or associated with) pyrethroid resistance, the larval stage-specific expressions of CYP9M10 and CYP4H34 genes are consistent with the following facts: the one lies in the laboratory selection of 4th instar larvae with permethrin during establishment of this strain (12); another comes from larval specific pyrethroid resistance which was greatly decreased by *in vivo* inhibition of P450 monooxygenases (11).

Further studies on resistance-associated cytochrome P450s

Although almost two decades has been passed since the first insect P450 gene was identified from the housefly (13), little is known for the regulatory mechanisms of insect P450 genes. It has been clarified that in *Drosophila*, insertion of a transposon (accord) on the upstream region of the structural gene is related to the up-regulation of Cyp6g1 that causes high levels of cross-resistance to DDT and imidacloprid. Such resistant fruit flies with the same mechanism were observed almost all over the world (14). Transposons or their fragmented traces have been identified near by P450 loci of other insects including housefly CYP6D1 and CYP6D3 (15) and anopheline CYP6Z1 (16). In these reports the inserted transposon are suspected as a possible cause of constitutively overexpressed P450 gene. Moreover, two other possible molecular mechanisms have been reported for the overproduction of enzyme that is associated with insecticide resistance. The one is trans-acting mutations that modulate P450 gene expression such as demonstrated with housefly CYP6A1 (17) and CYP6D1 (18). Another is gene amplification as observed in the carboxyl esterase genes of *Myzus persicae* (19) and *Cx. pipiens* complex (20).

Analyses of the genomic structures of CYP9M10 and CYP4H34 and the genetic factors correlated with their overexpressions will be needed to deduce responsible mutations for further studies. The identification of the P450 isoforms that catalyze the metabolisms of pyrethroid insecticides will facilitate the development of new synergists which enhance the effect of mosquitocides. Both genetic and biochemical approaches will assist the monitoring and management of insecticide-based *Culex* control programs.

Conclusions

Outstanding larval etofenprox resistance has developed in the natural populations of *Cx. p.* molestus and *Cx. p. pallens* in Japan. The resistance crosses to other pyrethroids with phenoxy-benzyl moiety. Both *kdr* and elevated P450 detoxification were involved in the larval pyrethroid-resistance mechanisms as major factors. Multiple P450 genes were overexpressing in etophenprox-resistant strains that are showing 10^3 level resistance, however, their overexpression patterns were not necessarily common to the resistant strains. Both transcription ratios (represented by R/S ratio) and absolute transcription levels (measured in contrast with a housekeeping gene) of CYP9M10 and CYP4H34 genes were extraordinarily high in JPP strain of *Cx. quinquefasciatus*.

Acknowledgment

This work was partly supported by Grant-in-Aids for Scientific Research of Emerging and Reemerging Infectious Diseases from the Ministry of Health, Labor and Welfare (H15-Shinko-18) and for Scientific Research from The Ministry of Education, Culture, Sports, Science and Technology-Japan (14770113, 17790281, 16380045, and 19580062).

References

1. Kawakami, Y. *Jpn. J. Sanit. Zool.* **1989**, 40, 217-220.
2. Hayes, E. B.; Komar N.; Nasci, R. S.; Montgomery, S. P.;O'Leary, D. R.; Campbell, G. L. *Emerg. Infect. Dis.* **2005**, 11: 1167-1173.
3. Hotta, S. *Med. Entomol. Zool.* **1998**, 49: 267-274.
4. Shono, T. *J. Pestic. Sci.* **2005**, 30: 319-320.
5. Kasai, S.; Shono, T.; Komahata, O.; Tsuda, Y.; Kobayashi, M.; Motoki, M.; Kashima, I.; Tanikawa, T.; Yoshida, M.; Tanaka, I.; Shinjo, G.; Hashinoto, T.; Ishikawa, T.; Takahashi, T.; Higa, Y.; Tomita, T. *J. Med. Entomol.* **2007**, 44, 822-829.
6. Asahina, S.; Yasutomi, K.; Noguchi, K. *Jpn. J. Sanit. Zool.* **1963**, 14, 167-175.
7. Shono, T; *J. Pestic. Sci.* **1985**, 10, 141-146.
8. Komagata, O.; Kasai, S.; Obara, I.; Motoyama, N.; Tanaka, I.; Kobayashi, M.; Yomita, T. *Med. Entomol. Zool.* **2008**, 59, 33-46.
9. Weerasinghe, I. S.; Kasai, S.; Shono, T. *J. Pestic. Sci.* **2001**, 26, 158-161.
10. Kasai, S.,; Weerasinghe, I. S.; Shono, T. Arch. *Insect Biochem. Physiol.* **1998**, 37, 47-56.
11. Hardstone, M.C.; Leichter, C.; Harrington, L.C.; Kasai, S.; Tomita, T.; Scott, J. G. *Pestic. Biochem. Physiol.* **2007**, 89, 175-184.
12. Amin, A. M.; Hemingway, J. *Bull. Ent. Res.* **1989**, 79, 361-366.
13. Feyereisen, R.; Koener, J. F.; Farnsworth, D. E.; Nebert, D. W.; *Proc. Natl. Acad. Sci. USA* **1989**, 86, 1465-1469.
14. Catania, F.; Kauer, M. O.; Daborn, P. J.; Yen, J. L.; ffrench-Constant, R. H.; Schlotterer, C. *Mol. Ecol.* **2004**, 13, 2491-2504.
15. Kasai, S.; Scott, J. G.; *Insect Mol. Biol.* **2001**, 10, 191-196.
16. Nikou, D.; Ranson, H.; Hemingway, J. *Gene* **2003**, 318, 91-102.
17. Carino, F. A.; Koener, J. F.; Plapp, J. F. W.; Feyereisen, R. *Insect Biochem. Mol. Biol.* **1994**, 24. 411-418.
18. Carino, F.; Koener, J. F.; Plapp, F. W. J.; Feyereisen, R. In *Molecular Mechanisms of Insecticide Resistance: Diversity Among Insects*, Mullin, C.A.; Scott, J.G. eds., **1992**, Vol. 505, pp. 31-40. Washington D.C., American Chemical Society.
19. Field, L. M.; Devonshire, A. L.; Forde, B. G.; *Biochem. J.* **1988**, 251, 309-312.
20. Mouches, C.; Pauplin, Y.; Agarwal, M.; Lemieux, L.; Herzog, M.; Abadon, M.; Beyssat-Arnaouty, V.; Hyrien, O.; de Saint Vincent, B. R.; Georghiou, G. P. *Proc. Natl. Acad. Sci. USA* **1990**, 87, 2574-2578.

Chapter 4

Vector Control for Prevention of Dengue

Current Status and Future Strategies

Tessa B. Knox and Thomas W. Scott

Department of Entomology, University of California, Davis, CA 95616

When implemented properly, vector control can be an effective strategy for preventing mosquito-borne disease. Yet dengue control failures continue to be the norm rather than the exception. Reliance on prescribed control strategies and targets continues despite a clear understanding that the complex dynamics of dengue virus transmission is inconsistent with universal efficacy. Promising advances in control technology are on the horizon, but it is unlikely these will be effective for use either in isolation or across all epidemiological situations. Locally-adaptive control strategies that combine available tools in a manner suitable for the particular situation will increase the uptake, efficacy, and impact of dengue vector control programs.

Widespread adoption of a locally-adaptive approach to dengue vector control will require a paradigm shift from current strategies (*1*). For vector control programs and personnel to effectively move from broadly-prescribed guidelines to autonomous decisions based on locally-derived information, vector control managers and public health personnel require clearer information about available tools (including advantages and limitations of each), the best combinations of tools, and the optimal timing and extent of application. In this chapter, we discuss what is required to support the move toward locally-adaptive dengue prevention strategies and why these will be more effective than universally applied programs. This is examined in the context of past and present experiences in utilizing vector control for reducing the burden of dengue.

The Global Problem of Dengue

Dengue is a major international public health concern. It is the most important arthropod-borne viral disease of humans in terms of both morbidity and mortality. The four related but distinct dengue viruses (DENV-1, DENV-2, DENV-3 and DENV-4) belong to the genus *Flavivirus* (family Flaviviridae), and are maintained in disease endemic settings in a human to mosquito transmission cycle. Sylvatic cycles with transmission to monkeys have been documented in Asia and Africa (*2*), but do not appear to be necessary for maintenance of the human-mosquito cycle. In humans, infections can range from asymptomatic to mild undifferentiated fever, classical dengue fever or dengue hemorrhagic fever (DHF). The latter is the most severe and without adequate hospital care can result in death.

Over 2.5 billion people in tropical and subtropical areas of the world are at risk of dengue virus infection; an estimated 50 million infections and half a million cases of DHF result each year (*3*). Dengue viruses are endemic to South-East Asia, the Western Pacific, the Americas, the eastern Mediterranean and Africa. The majority of disease burden is in low- to middle- income countries in the first three regions (*4, 5*),

Dengue exacts an enormous toll on the economies of affected communities, although the financial costs involved are difficult to measure. Direct costs include that of hospitalization and intensive care for acutely ill patients. Disrupted earning potential due to illness or the need to look after a sick family member often results even when hospitalization is not necessary. In South-East Asia, losses per case of dengue or DHF were estimated at US$12.39, with a corresponding loss in disability-adjusted life years (DALYs) of 0.39 per 1000 population (*6*). For Thailand alone, an estimated financial loss of US$61 per family in 2001 exceeded the annual monthly income. The associated loss of 0.43 DALYs per 1000 population was in the same order of magnitude as for malaria, meningitis, hepatitis and the tropical cluster diseases (*7*). Similar estimates were made for DALYs lost to dengue in Puerto Rico from 1984 to 1994 (*8*). The high cost of vector control activities in addition to possible lost revenue due to reduced tourism contribute to the economic burden. Other indirect costs related to social disruption resulting from large epidemics of 'flu-like' illness may also be significant.

The World Health Assembly designated the control and prevention of dengue a high priority in 1993, and a global strategy against dengue was adopted in 1995 (*9*). However, due to the complex epidemiological dynamics of dengue, there is a lack of effective strategies to combat the disease (Table I). At present, there is no clinical treatment for dengue and a vaccine is still under development. Consequently, the only viable option for alleviating the burden of dengue involves reducing contact between humans and potentially infectious vectors, mainly by suppressing populations of the principal global dengue vector, *Aedes aegypti*.

The geographic distribution, incidence and severity of dengue disease have increased over the past few decades as a result of numerous complex factors, many of which are associated with increasing populations of *Ae. aegypti.* Changes in vector distribution and abundance have been linked to major global human demographic changes; uncontrolled increases in human population and urbanization have resulted in absent or deficient water and sanitation infrastructure and have necessitated the storage of water. Changing consumer habits have increased the production of solid waste (i.e., discarded plastic items, used automobile tires), which increase the availability of potential mosquito development sites for vectors. Increased air travel by humans has facilitated rapid transportation of the dengue viruses between population centers of the tropics. Although *Ae. albopictus* has been incriminated in some outbreaks (*10-12*), the anthropophilic blood feeding habitat, frequency of human contact, and close proximity to human hosts make *Ae. aegypti* an extremely efficient vector for dengue viruses (*13, 14*). Many of these characteristics also complicate vector control (Table II).

Further increases in dengue morbidity and mortality are inevitable unless changes are made to the way we conduct control. Deteriorating public health infrastructure is placing more of an emphasis on emergency, reactive disease control rather than on the implementation of preventative measures (*15*). Ineffective mosquito and dengue surveillance and control practices in the vast majority of dengue-endemic countries exacerbates the situation. Some predict that global warming will increase the public health impact of dengue although this remains controversial (*16-19*). Examination of past vector control successes and failures will help to determine what is needed to face current and future challenges to the prevention of dengue.

Table I. Why is dengue so problematic?

Characteristics	*Implications for Control*
The majority of transmission occurs in developing countries	There are limited resources and infrastructure for prevention and control
Distribution is widespread and increasing, and is no longer confined to urban areas	Virus is introduced into susceptible (seronaïve) populations and areas where there is limited experience and capacity to conduct control
Transmission of all four serotypes is increasing worldwide	Increasing incidence and severity of disease put a strain on health systems and reduce capacity to implement control
Transmission is not uniform	Large and rapid outbreaks that occur periodically, seasonally, and vary between years and regions may overwhelm health facilities
Complex immunological dynamics due to four antigenically-distinct serotypes	Despite long-term homologous immunity, antibody dependent immune enhancement may increase the chance of DHF during a secondary infection. A tetravalent vaccine protective against all serotypes is required
Infection causes a continuum of disease, with a high inapparent to apparent ratio	Diagnosis may be difficult and case detection is not always a reliable indicator of transmission, thus the use of case data for guiding control is limited
Determinants of DHF pathogenesis are incompletely understood	Difficult to target protective measures at individuals most at risk of severe disease
3 – 14 days incubation between infection and development of symptoms	Although effective for management/treatment of individual cases, anti-virals may not be a practical method for community protection
No rapid, cheap, and efficient way to determine serotype-specific susceptibility of human populations	Based on currently available methodologies it is impractical to monitor transmission and implement control based on serological surveillance
No specific treatment	Because there is no cure, viraemic individuals continue to contribute to transmission

Table II. Why is *Aedes aegypti* so problematic?

Characteristics	*Implications for Control*
Anthropophilic: feed preferentially and frequently on humans	High contact rates with humans mean that vector population densities may need to be reduced to very low levels before significant reductions in transmission result
Endophilic: rest indoors	Outdoor spraying (e.g., using truck-mounted sprayers) is not effective. Home-based techniques that kill mosquitoes where they rest and at the primary point of human infection are more appropriate (i.e., indoor residual spraying, insecticide-treated materials, space spraying)
Endophagic: feed indoors	Interventions directed toward the indoor, intradomicile environment and that prevent contact with humans may be effective (e.g., personal repellents, indoor insecticide-treated materials)
Diurnal feeding: bite during the day	Blood-seeking during times of high human activity mean that vector population densities may need to be reduced to very low levels before significant reductions in transmission result Bednets may be a less effective means of personal protection than for night-biting mosquitoes
Larval habitats generally found in close proximity to human habitation	Water intentionally stored in or around household in some areas will restrict the applicability of source reduction activities to non-essential containers (e.g., discards)
Larval habitats are diverse	Source reduction may deflect gravid females to alternate oviposition sites
Dispersal by flight of adult mosquitoes generally limited to <100 meters	Most dispersal of virus occurs through viraemic host movement. This should be considered when determining the spatial distribution of control activities
Distribution is widespread and is increasing	Expansion into previously uncolonized areas means that the capacity required to conduct control activities (e.g., experience and resources) may be lacking

History of *Aedes aegypti* Control

There are a number of historical examples of *Ae. aegypti* control that resulted in elimination or significant reduction of human disease. Following confirmation of *Ae. aegypti* as the vector of yellow fever virus, a large scale mosquito control program was initiated in Havana, Cuba in the early 1900s. Championed by Major William C. Gorgas, this program mainly involved elimination of larval habitats. Eradication of yellow fever - as well as significant reductions in malaria incidence - resulted within 8 months (*20*). Gorgas subsequently initiated a similar program to protect workers involved in the construction of the Panama Canal. An intensive vector control campaign using source reduction, larviciding and adulticiding resulted in striking reductions in yellow fever cases, thereby permitting completion of the canal.

Control successes in Brazil in the 1930s led to the *Aedes aegypti* eradication program of the 1940s to 1960s, which was spearheaded by the Pan American Health Organization. Large paramilitary, vertically-structured programs proved successful, and eradication of *Ae. aegypti* resulted in all but four of 27 countries (*21, 22*). The approach taken involved meticulous inspection of potential larval development sites and their treatment with the organic insecticide dichloro-diphenyl-trichloroethane (DDT). Dengue and yellow fever transmission throughout Central and South America was largely extinguished.

When resistance to DDT rapidly emerged in the late 1960s (*23*) and other political and logistical problems resulted in interruptions to control programs, *Ae. aegypti* began to re-infest areas from which it had been eliminated (*21, 24*). As the distribution of *Ae. aegypti* expanded, eradication was progressively less plausible, and the eradication effort was unofficially abandoned in the early 1970s. Dengue and yellow fever transmission returned or intensified, and almost all of the countries previously declared *Ae. aegypti*-free were re-colonized by this species.

In recent years, significant reductions in dengue transmission have resulted from anti-*Ae. aegypti* activities in Cuba, Singapore and Vietnam. Eradication of *Ae. aegypti* and dengue was almost accomplished in Cuba during the early 1980s by using larval source reduction and adult mosquito control (*25*). However, success was difficult to sustain due to a number of factors including a breakdown in control activities (*26*). Singapore has maintained very low *Ae. aegypti* populations for over 35 years using mainly source reduction with public involvement through education and law enforcement (*27, 28*). Despite low vector densities, a resurgence of dengue occurred in 1986 and high transmission levels have persisted since (*27-29*). This has been attributed in part to changes in human infection patterns and immunity, such as increased transmission outside the home and reduced herd immunity in older age groups that are at greater risk of developing clinical dengue (*28, 30*). Increasing viral introductions by those travelling from other dengue-receptive areas and an emphasis on case-reactive control also contribute to the problem in Singapore (*28*). In Vietnam, community-based source reduction coupled with targeted distribution of larvivorous *Mesocyclops* copepods has been successful in eradicating *Ae. aegypti* from localities in northern and central regions (*31*). This has resulted in reductions in reported dengue morbidity and mortality rates compared to the surrounding areas, although actual dengue infection and seroconversion rates are unknown. Sustainability assessments are currently being conducted and the method was recently expanded into the southern Mekong Delta region of Vietnam, where the majority of dengue transmission occurs (P. A. Ryan, personal communication).

Lessons Learned

These examples of successful vector control indicate that while reductions in dengue can been achieved via reduction in vector populations, they are difficult to sustain. Even where long-term suppression of *Ae. aegypti* populations is achieved, low or absent transmission will not necessarily persist. It is possible that sustained low entomological indices may increase the force of dengue transmission (*30*), although this has yet to be definitively proven and warrants further investigation. With few exceptions, vector control programs have been unsuccessful at long-term suppression or prevention of dengue.

The reasons behind the poor success rate and lack of sustainability of vector control are complex (*32*). They include inadequate or misapplied vector control tools, breakdowns in public health infrastructure, insufficient resources and poor political support for control efforts. The complexity of dengue vector and transmission dynamics results in a lack of understanding of crucial spatial and temporal heterogeneities (*1*). Failure to consider the ecology of transmission and other relevant site-specific factors limits the effectiveness of dengue control programs.

The World Health Organization has promoted the use of traditional larval prevalence indices for setting control aims and priorities. It is assumed that a universal baseline index of fewer than five *Ae. aegypti* larvae-positive containers per 100 houses will confer community protection against dengue transmission. This index, which was originally devised for the yellow fever eradication efforts of last century, assigns each larval-positive container an equal value. However, the relationship between immature and adult populations is poorly defined and will vary depending on a multiplicity of intrinsic and extrinsic conditions. Indeed, differential productivity of adult *Ae. aegypti* both between and within containers of a particular type has been clearly demonstrated (*33-35*).

Specification of such programmatic aims is based on an assumption inherent to vector control: that there is a positive relationship between mosquito populations and risk of pathogen transmission (*36*). Although there have been attempts to empirically link entomological surveillance data with dengue transmission, reports have been variable. There are numerous examples of dengue transmission occurring when entomological indices are low (*27, 28, 37-39*). Conversely, an absence of local dengue transmission may occur when vector densities are high and dengue virus introductions occur (*40*). Clearly, the complex nature of dengue transmission means that such universally-prescribed control goals are inappropriate, and there have been numerous calls to abandon this approach (*41-44*).

In the past, emergency dengue control interventions relied almost exclusively on space spraying using thermal fogging or ultra light volume

(ULV) delivery of chemicals via truck- or airplane-mounted apparatus. This had the advantage of high visibility such that residents in areas under treatment were aware of control efforts on the part of the health authorities. This approach failed to take into consideration the indoor resting and avoidance behavior of female *Ae. aegypti* (*43*), which rendered outdoor-focused spraying largely ineffective. Although some control success resulted (*45*), effectiveness was for the most part short-lived. As irrefutable reports of control failures mounted, it became apparent that truck-mounted or aerial application of insecticides was largely ineffective (*46-49*) except in places where house construction allowed penetration of insecticide into the home. Backpack ULV aspirators were increasingly used for indoor space spraying, although broad-scale outdoor spraying is still conducted in some areas.

Past dengue control programs have been criticized for failing to consider the social and ecological factors that influence effectiveness (*48, 50*). Some argue that the vertically-structured, universal approach taken in the yellow fever eradication era (and currently applied to some extent in Singapore and Cuba) is inappropriate for most dengue-endemic countries. During the 1980s, there was a shift in emphasis from 'top down' vertically structured approaches to 'bottom up' community-based activities (*48, 51*). This addressed the need for integrated strategies incorporating health education and community ownership in order to encourage householder and neighborhood participation. The "top down" component was considered essential in the beginning phases of a campaign, with progressive emphasis on community involvement to secure sustainability (*48*). Such an approach combining active surveillance, emergency response, case management, and community-based *Ae. aegypti* control, was widely accepted and became the basis for the WHO global strategy for dengue prevention and control (*51*). Similar regional declarations were presented in the Americas and the Asia Pacific region and numerous countries implemented control programs centered on active community participation (*50, 52*). Although there is only weak evidence that community-based programs are effective and no examples of control success arising from actions initiated solely at the community level (*53*), general consensus is that some level of community involvement is imperative to secure effective and sustainable *Ae. aegypti* control.

The traditional reliance on single intervention methods and broad-sweeping guidelines, a lack of consideration of societal factors and poor involvement of non-health sectors has hindered the development of a conceptual and factual foundation for locally-devised integrated strategies (*1*). Yet it is obvious based on past experience that consideration of local conditions is imperative if more effective control programs are to be developed. This will require a major paradigm shift, whereby vector control departments or personnel use location-specific information to tailor strategies that are epidemiologically, ecologically and socially appropriate. Consistent monitoring and evaluation to assess the ongoing effect of intervention activities, and to adjust strategies in response to changes in vector and human populations over time, will be critical to any adaptive disease prevention system. In order to determine what is required to support such a shift, the current situation for dengue vector control must be examined.

Current Status of Dengue Control

Although there are inherent limitations associated with vector control, reducing the density of dengue vectors remains the only viable option for preventing and controlling dengue transmission to humans. Despite decades of research attention (*4, 32, 54, 55*), there is still no licensed, publicly-available vaccine against dengue. Progress has been hampered by (a) the need to develop a tetravalent vaccine effective against all four dengue serotypes due to the possibility of immune-enhancement, (b) a lack of a reliable animal model for DHF and the poor growth of dengue viruses in cell culture (*55*), and (c) a general lack of financial support for dengue vaccine research (*54*). Clinical trials of vaccine candidates are ongoing and it is reasonable to expect that a suitable vaccine will eventually be available (*32, 56*). It is possible, however, that the resultant vaccine will be of restricted utility in dengue-endemic countries due to accessibility limitations (*57*). For instance, other arboviral diseases such as Japanese encephalitis and yellow fever persist despite the availability of effective vaccines (*58*). Promising antiviral therapeutics may be on the horizon (*59*), but these are likely to have a limited effect on overall transmission among human populations. It is likely that mosquito control will remain a vital component of dengue control initiatives even after the advent of effective, commercially-available dengue therapeutics or vaccines.

Vector control currently comprises the core of almost all operational dengue control programs worldwide. In 1994, the Pan American Health Organization declared the eradication of *Ae. aegypti* an unattainable goal (*60*), and adjusted to a focus on cost-effective utilization of limited resources in order to reduce vector populations to levels at which they are no longer of significant public health importance (*15, 60*). In 1993, the World Health Assembly officially designated dengue control and prevention a high priority, and in 1995 a global strategy was drafted that advocated the use of new surveillance and control tools in combination with intersectoral involvement, better training of field staff, and community participation (*9*). In 2002, the Executive Board of the WHO passed a resolution that, among other items, recognized "that prevention or reduction of dengue viral transmission entirely depends on control of the mosquito vector *Aedes aegypti* and, to a lesser extent, *Ae. albopictus* and other secondary vector species" (*61*). Moreover, it stated that "dengue vector-control programmes have had considerable success in the past, but that sustained suppression of vector populations today largely depends on the collective actions and behaviors of all members of affected communities to prevent breeding of *Ae. aegypti*". In line with this, a newly-formulated Asia-Pacific Dengue Partnership framework also relies on dengue prevention and reduction through vector control, with a focus on householder and community participation and mobilization.

Control programs for *Ae. aegypti* vary worldwide, largely as a result of country-specific economic constraints and availability of vector control products. The majority of countries document a combined strategy of immature vector surveillance, chemical/biological treatment or destruction of larval habitats, and either routine or emergency reactive application of ULV space sprays against adult mosquitoes. In reality, limited resources mean that health ministries are unwilling to commit resources except for requisite emergency mosquito control interventions in response to epidemics (*62*). Entomological surveillance usually plays no significant role except when monitoring for incursions of exotic species or during eradication programs. Most endemic countries have poorly-defined control goals, and surveillance data are rarely used for epidemic risk predictions. Most dengue control programs are currently ill-equipped to develop and maintain sustained community participation strategies, such as source reduction (*63*). Increasingly, control programs are faced with the challenge of insecticide-resistant *Ae. aegypti* populations.

Aedes aegypti control programs around the world are, for the most part, failing to secure reductions in disease. In most dengue-endemic countries, human populations are plagued by a multiplicity of infectious diseases, and resources available for vector control are rarely what is needed for sustained disease prevention. Although history provides numerous examples of vector control successes, the current ecological, epidemiologic and political situation presents unique challenges. It is clear that we need to develop ways to use the limited vector control resources to more effectively reduce dengue burden.

The Future of Dengue Prevention

Preventing the transmission of dengue viruses requires either (a) reductions in *Ae. aegypti* abundance in order to reduce the frequency of contact with humans, (b) prevention of contact between *Ae. aegypti* and humans using barriers or deterrents, (c) alteration of the age structure of *Ae. aegypti* populations to favor younger mosquitoes that have a lower chance of being infective and transmitting virus, (d) reduction of the susceptibility and transmission potential of individual *Ae. aegypti* or (e) artificial enhancement of human herd immunity (such as through vaccination) to reduce the probability of transmission. The majority of currently available control tools target (a), although all of these approaches are currently under investigation. Many have been reviewed in detail elsewhere (*1, 62, 64*) and some will be discussed in subsequent chapters. Serious consideration must be given to what is required to support the further development of these tools, and to ensure their effective application in locally-adaptive disease prevention strategies.

Accounting for Heterogeneities

Dengue transmission involves vector, virus and host interactions that are affected by intrinsic and extrinsic factors (*65*). *Aedes aegypti* abundance and capacity for transmission are modulated by environmental variables such as temperature and host associations including the availability of larval development sites. Virus transmission is influenced by susceptibility of the human population (i.e., herd immunity), contact with competent mosquito vectors, and introduction of virus. As a result, the quantitative relationship between *Ae. aegypti* density and dengue transmission risk is dynamic and complex, and exhibits both spatial and temporal variability (*36*).

Characterizing sources of variation - such as the subset of humans that contribute disproportionately to transmission or are at a highest risk of serious disease - may help to identify key targets for control. For instance, observed disparities in immature *Ae. aegypti* populations sustained in different aquatic habitats lead to the notion that directing larval control to highly productive containers will enhance the effectiveness of vector control programs (*33, 66*). Such targeted control is the subject of a current TDR multi-country study. Although a theoretically sound concept, numerous other factors require consideration. For instance, will the removal or treatment of a subset of containers encourage oviposition in remaining containers, or will it encourage the dispersal of gravid (and potentially infectious) females as they seek alternative oviposition sites (*67*)?

Locally tailored strategies can account for site-by-site and temporal variation in vector populations and virus transmission. Tools are required that support the formulation of such flexible strategies. A user-friendly computer program for simulating *Ae. aegypti* populations and dengue transmission is currently being developed by the Innovative Vector Control Consortium (*68*). It is anticipated that the model will help public health personnel and vector control program managers in dengue-receptive areas explore the relative impact of interventions simulated under local conditions, in order to formulate appropriate control strategies. The computer model will be a supplement to the Dengue Decision Support System under development by the same group (*64*). These will assist policy makers and program managers in the effective use of available resources by providing relevant information and data on disease incidence, vector populations and insecticide resistance. In this way, resources may be allocated preferentially to these targets in order to optimize the cost, timeliness and efficacy of control programs.

Adult Surveillance and Control

Vector surveillance efforts for dengue generally focus on immature aquatic stages of *Ae. aegypti.* There is, however, an overall poor relationship between immature and adult populations (especially for larvae) (*35, 44, 69-71*), and associations with virus transmission (Morrison, Scott and Kochel, University of California (Davis) and Naval Medical Research Centre Detachment (Iquitos): Unpublished data). Even though assessment of adult populations is preferable given their direct role in virus transmission, most programs focus surveillance efforts on immature mosquitoes due to the lack of practical and accurate tools for monitoring adults. *Aedes aegypti* is generally a low abundance mosquito that is difficult to catch in traps (Jones et al. 2003). Development of a cost-effective and practical method for estimating adult *Ae. aegypti* densities should be a priority (*62*). Collection of adults would also offer the opportunity to assay for virus-infected mosquitoes.

Control efforts generally focus on larvae except during epidemics, when emergency interventions often target adult *Ae. aegypti*. Although the impact of adulticidal activities have generally been short-lived (*46, 50, 72, 73*) and the majority of programs that have relied primarily on eliminating adult mosquitoes have failed (*48, 74*), we argue there is still an important role for adult control. Indeed, we caution against focusing control solely on the immature stages; if coverage is incomplete – which is generally the case due to the propensity of *Ae. aegypti* to exploit available larval development sites – the transmission potential of resulting adult populations may be enhanced (*75, 76*).

Although development of operationally- and cost-effective adult surveillance and control tools should be a priority (*1, 62*), it is likely that strategies assessing and targeting multiple life stages will be more effective than those that affect a single stage. The effectiveness of adulticidal approaches should be evaluated in comparison to, as well as in combination with, strategies that target immature stages in order to determine the most effective approach under different field situations.

Proactive Versus Reactive Intervention

The shift from the eradication paradigm of the 1940s – 1970s to a focus on reducing vector populations and disease to levels at which they are of no public health significance has revealed a number of unknowns (*1, 36*). Namely, what constitutes "public health significance" and how does this concept change through time and space? How should control goals be defined, and what constitutes a control failure or success? What vector surveillance data should be collected and how can it be best used to inform control activities such that interventions can be altered in response to changing conditions? Clearly, empirical data is required to support the formulation of realistic and epidemiologically-relevant vector control goals. Failure to reach set goals may have negative repercussions, both in terms of continued disease and future political – and hence financial and logistical support – for ongoing control programs.

Due to limited resources, the majority of dengue-endemic countries rely largely on passive rather than active surveillance systems (*61*) such that practices are heavily skewed toward reactive emergency measures. In theory, a major shift in resources allocation from reactive to proactive vector interventions will improve the outcome of control programs (*64*). This would be based on situation-specific combinations of proactive vector surveillance and control with pathogen and disease surveillance, and include reactive emergency vector control as required in response to epidemic transmission. It is unlikely that significant resources will be devoted to proactive control in areas where there are budgetary or other resource constraints without strong governmental support. Justification for proactive control must then be made on the basis of economic viability. Also requiring consideration is the situation in which the control program is successful and dengue is decreased to such low levels as to no longer be of public health significance. As with the *Ae. aegypti* eradication campaign of earlier years, it is likely that funds necessary for proactive control will be funneled off to other existing or emerging diseases of relatively higher public health importance.

An alternative to government-directed proactive intervention lies in shifting the onus of control to householders. A '*casa segura*' or safe house approach has been proposed, in which the home environment is the focus of anti-*Ae. aegypti* activities (*1, 64*). This capitalizes on the peridomestic nature of *Ae. aegypti* by directing control to its primary resting, biting and larval development location: people's homes. This approach is supported by the advent of long-lasting insecticide-treated materials, which have proven effective against malaria in many parts of the world, and also against *Ae. aegypti* in southeast Asia (*77-79*) and the Americas (*80, 81*). Use of such materials, which have thus far been formulated into bednets, curtains and container covers, offers a proactive approach to dengue prevention that depends on householder involvement. On a smaller scale, personal barriers such as repellent sprays may also confer some protection against biting *Ae. aegypti*. Expecting householders to contribute to the financing, implementation and maintenance of such control measures is justified on the basis that a certain amount of household expenditure in many developing countries may already be devoted to anti-mosquito activities. In Thailand, householders spend US$2 – 25 per year per household on insecticides, which constitutes a greater amount than was spent on organized mosquito control (*82*). This indicates a significant market for safe and effective personal protection tools which may require minimal top-down involvement. Provision of clear and accurate information on the most suitable methods to apply is imperative to the success of a "*case segura*" approach.

Integrated Targets and Tools

Control activities targeting *Ae. aegypti* have the potential to significantly reduce other non-target vector populations and diseases. Source reduction may reduce populations of container-breeding vector and nuisance mosquitoes such as *Ae. albopictus*, *Aedes notoscriptus*, and *Culex pipiens*. Anti-*Ae. aegypti* activities will contribute to a reduction in yellow fever and chikungunya transmission and, as demonstrated during interventions at the Panama Canal, may lead to the reduction of other arthropod-borne diseases such as malaria. The potential effect of expanding the goals and targets of a dengue control program to include other vector-borne diseases needs to be evaluated. In this way, the public health impact of anti-dengue programs can be leveraged by reducing overall disease, increasing uptake and sustainability of the program, and ultimately alleviating the strain on health systems such that resources are freed for the control of other diseases. Control measures that kill nuisance pests as well as vectors will be more appealing to households and may enhance community uptake and participation (*62*).

A fundamental observation in dengue prevention is that there is no one method or approach that is effective in all situations (*36*). Certain methods applicable in one area may not be feasible in another. For instance, biological control with *Mesocyclops* is useful in Vietnam because restrictions limit the registration and use of chemical control agents in water for human consumption. However, the utility of this approach may be restricted to areas where large containers predominate and the social structure is amenable to a community-based programmatic structure (*83*). Experience with lymphatic filariasis indicates that drug administration along with vector control will have a greater impact that either approach alone (*84-86*). It is likely that greater reductions in dengue transmission will result from a combination of immunization and vector control strategies than through using any method in isolation (*1*). A dengue vaccine will prevent dengue whereas vector control may confer protection against several pathogens. Thus, even in the advent of an effective dengue vaccine and 100% coverage of an at-risk human population, it is likely that *Ae. aegypti* vector control will remain an important component of public health programs. The right combination of control tools can increase the likelihood of control success and may improve the sustainability of public health and vector control programs (*1*).

Sustainability

A number of promising dengue vector control programs have failed to achieve long term disease reductions due to waning political commitment and lack of community support (*87*). If vector control success was sufficient to ensure programmatic sustainability, we would not have witnessed the resurgence in dengue following the breakdown in yellow fever eradication efforts. Even in the case of long-term, effective vector control in Singapore, reductions in dengue transmission were difficult to maintain (*28*). Yet sustainability is a key focus of the global dengue prevention strategy (*88*), and it is clear that ongoing activities are required if significant reductions in dengue are to be achieved (*62*).

The strengthening of intersectoral management structures in Cuba has been shown to improve coordination of community-based anti-dengue activities, and lead to increased community knowledge and practices and ultimately more effective vector control (*89*). Although there are numerous examples of failed top-down approaches to *Ae. aegypti* control (*73, 90-92*), reliance solely on the community to assume responsibility for vector control is risky (*62, 72*).

Towards Locally-Adaptive Dengue Prevention

Locally-adaptive dengue prevention will facilitate the formulation of strategies relevant to the local conditions of respective dengue-receptive areas. Due to variations in availability, means of application, and resources among localities we expect options to be limited from one place to another. Formulation of appropriate strategies must consider the public health and vector control infrastructure of the area. Now that we realize that universally prescribed control goals and strategies are inappropriate due to the diversity of factors that affect transmission, attention can be focused on developing, evaluating and applying control tools and strategies that will be appropriate to the given situation. In order to support such a shift in the approach to dengue control, we view the following as priority areas for attention.

- Characterize sources of spatial and temporal variation in vector populations and virus transmission in order to identify the dimensions of risk and transmission, identify potential targets for control, and provide a theoretical framework to support locally-adaptive dengue prevention strategies.

- Focus on the development of *Ae. aegypti* adult population monitoring and control tools, and assess the effectiveness of these independently and in combination with tools targeting immature stages in a variety of field settings.
- Evaluate the theoretical impact of differential resource allocation between proactive and reactive vector control for different areas, including an assessment of shifting the onus of control to householders.
- Investigate the impact of a combination of vector control and other disease reduction tools on *Ae. aegypti* and other local non-target vector/nuisance populations, and incidence of dengue and other diseases, in order to leverage available resources for overall disease reduction.
- Promote the formulation of strategies that integrate top-down and bottom-up involvement in order to ensure sustainability and uptake of disease control activities across all sociopolitical situations.

References

1. Scott, T. W.; Morrison, A. C. In *Vector-Borne Diseases: Understanding the Environmental, Human Health, and Ecological Connections*, Lemon, S. M.; Sparling, P. F.; Hamburg, M. A.; Relman, D. A.; Coffnes, E. R.; Mack, A., Eds. The National Academies Press: Washington, DC, 2008; pp 132-149.
2. Rodhain, F.; Rosen, L. In *Dengue and Dengue Hemorrhagic Fever*, New York, 1997; pp 45-60.
3. *Report of the Scientific Working Group meeting on Dengue*; Special Programme for Research & Training in Tropical Diseases (TDR): Geneva, Switzerland, 1-5 October 2006.
4. Guzman, M. G.; Kouri, G. *Lancet Infect. Dis.* **2002,** *2*, 33-42.
5. Renganathan, E.; Parks, W.; Lloyd, L.; Nathan, M. B.; Hosein, E.; Odugleh, A.; Clark, G. G.; Gubler, D. J.; Prasittisuk, C.; Palmer, K. *Dengue Bulletin* **2003,** *27*, 6-12.
6. Shepard, D. S.; Suaya, J. A.; Halstead, S. B.; Nathan, M. B.; Gubler, D. J.; Mahoney, R. T.; Wang, D. N.; Meltzer, M. I. *Vaccine* **2004,** *22*, 1275-1280.
7. Clark, D. V.; Mammen, M. P., Jr.; Nisalak, A.; Puthimethee, V.; Endy, T. P. *Am. J. Trop. Med. Hyg.* **2005,** *72*, 786-791.
8. Meltzer, M. I.; Rigau-Perez, J. G.; Clark, G. G.; Reiter, P.; Gubler, D. J. *Am. J. Trop. Med. Hyg.* **1998,** *59*, 265-271.
9. *Report of the consultation on: key issues in dengue vector control toward the operationalization of a global strategy.* CTD/FIL(DEN)/IC/96.1; World Health Organization: Geneva, Switzerland, 1995.
10. Effler, P. V.; Pang, L.; Kitsutani, P.; Vorndam, V.; Nakata, M.; Ayers, T.; Elm, J.; Tom, T.; Reiter, P.; Rigau-Perez, J. G.; Hayes, J. M.; Mills, K.; Napier, M.; Clark, G. G.; Gubler, D. J. *Emerg. Infect. Dis.* **2005,** *11*, 742-749.

11. Fontenille, D.; Toto, J. C. *Emerg. Infect. Dis.* **2001,** *7*, 1066-1067.
12. Metselaar, D.; Grainger, C. R.; Oei, K. G.; Reynolds, D. G.; Pudney, M.; Leake, C. J.; Tukei, P. M.; D'Offay, R. M.; Simpson, D. I. *Bull. World Health Organ.* **1980,** *58*, 937-943.
13. Scott, T. W.; Clark, G. G.; Lorenz, L. H.; Amerasinghe, P. H.; Reiter, P.; Edman, J. D. *J. Med. Entomol.* **1993,** *30*, 94-99.
14. Scott, T. W.; Naksathit, A.; Day, J. F.; Kittayapong, P.; Edman, J. D. *Am. J. Trop. Med. Hyg.* **1997,** *57*, 235-239.
15. Gubler, D. J. *Bull. Pan. Am. Health Organ.* **1989,** *23*, 397-404.
16. Hales, S.; de Wet, N.; Maindonald, J.; Woodward, A. *Lancet* **2002,** *360*, 830-834.
17. Jetten, T. H.; Focks, D. A. *Am. J. Trop. Med. Hyg.* **1997,** *57*, 285-297.
18. Patz, J. A.; Martens, W. J.; Focks, D. A.; Jetten, T. H. *Environ. Health Perspect.* **1998,** *106*, 147-153.
19. Stern, N., The economics of climate change: the Stern review. In *Cabinet Office - HM Treasury*, London, 2007.
20. Reeves, W. C. *Am. J. Trop. Med. Hyg.* **1980,** *29*, 1-10.
21. Schliessmann, D. J.; Calheiros, L. B. *Mosq. News* **1974,** *34*, 1-9.
22. Soper, F. L. *Amer. J. Pub. Health* **1963,** *53*, 7-16.
23. Brown, A. W.; Pal, R. *Public Health Pap.* **1971,** *38*, 1-491.
24. Reeves, W. C. *Recrudescence of arthropod-borne virus diseases in the Americas;* Scientific Publication No. 238; Pan American Health Organization: Washington, DC, 1972.
25. Kouri, G. P.; Guzman, M. G.; Bravo, J. R.; Triana, C. *Bull. World Health Organ.* **1989,** *67*, 375-380.
26. Kouri, G.; Guzman, M. G.; Valdes, L.; Carbonel, I.; del Rosario, D.; Vazquez, S.; Laferte, J.; Delgado, J.; Cabrera, M. V. *Emerg. Infect. Dis.* **1998,** *4*, 89-92.
27. Chan, K. L. *Singapore's dengue haemorrhagic fever control program: a case study on the successful control of* Aedes aegypti *and* Aedes albopictus *using mainly environmental measures as a part of integrated vector control*; Tokyo, Japan, 1985.
28. Ooi, E. E.; Goh, K. T.; Gubler, D. J. *Emerg. Infect. Dis.* **2006,** *12*, 887-893.
29. Ooi, E. E.; Hart, T. J.; Tan, H. C.; Chan, S. H. *Lancet* **2001,** *357*, 685-686.
30. Egger, J. R.; Ooi, E. E.; Kelly, D. W.; Woolhouse, M. E.; Davies, C. R.; Coleman, P. G. *Bull. World Health Organ.* **2008,** *86*, 187-196.
31. Kay, B.; Nam, V. S. *Lancet* **2005,** *365*, 613-617.
32. Halstead, S. B. *Dengue Bulletin* **2000,** *24*, 60-70.
33. Focks, D. A.; Alexander, N. *Multicountry study of Aedes aegypti pupal productivity survey methodology: findings and recommendations*; TDR/IRM/DEN/06.1; UNICEF/UNDP/World Bank/WHO Special Programme for Research and Training in Tropical Diseases: Geneva, Switzerland, 2006.
34. Knox, T. B. Optimising surveillance of immature *Aedes aegypti* in Vietnam. PhD thesis, University of Queensland, Brisbane, Australia, 2007.
35. Morrison, A. C.; Astete, H.; Chapilliquen, F.; Ramirez-Prada, C.; Diaz, G.; Getis, A.; Gray, K.; Scott, T. W. *J. Med. Entomol.* **2004,** *41*, 502-510.

36. Scott, T. W.; Morrison, A. C. In *Ecological Aspects for Application of Genetically Modified Mosquitoes*, Takken, W.; Scott, T. W., Eds. Kluwer Academic Publishers: Dordrecht, the Netherlands, 2004; pp 187-206.
37. Kay, B. H.; Barker-Hudson, P.; Hapgood, G. D.; McCurley, J. O.; Lyons, G. C.; Ives, W. *Gen. Appl. Entomol.* **1987,** *19*, 1-10.
38. Kuno, G. In *Dengue and Dengue Hemorrhagic Fever*, Gubler, D. J.; Kuno, G., Eds. CAB International: New York, 1997; pp 61-88.
39. Reiter, P. In *Dengue: A Worldwide Problem, a Common Strategy*, Halstead, S. B.; Gomez-Dantes, H., Eds. Ediciones Copilco: Mexico City, Mexico, 1992; pp 41-48.
40. Tewari, S. C.; Thenmozhi, V.; Katholi, C. R.; Manavalan, R.; Munirathinam, A.; Gajanana, A. *Trop. Med. Int. Health* **2004,** *9*, 499-507.
41. Focks, D. A. *A review of entomological sampling methods and indicators for dengue vectors*; TDR/IDE/Den/03.1; Special Programme for Research and Training in Tropical Diseases: Geneva, Switzerland, 2003.
42. Focks, D. A.; Chadee, D. D. *Am. J. Trop. Med. Hyg.* **1997,** *56*, 159-167.
43. Reiter, P.; Gubler, D. J. In *Dengue and Dengue Hemorrhagic Fever*, Gubler, D. J.; Kuno, G., Eds. CAB International: New York 1997; pp 425-462.
44. Tun-Lin, W.; Kay, B. H.; Barnes, A.; Forsyth, S. *Am. J. Trop. Med. Hyg.* **1996,** *54*, 543-547.
45. Gratz, N. G. *Annu. Rev. Entomol.* **1999,** *44*, 51-75.
46. Castle, T.; Amador, M.; Rawlins, S.; Figueroa, J. P.; Reiter, P. *Rev. Panam. Salud Publica* **1999,** *5*, 100-105.
47. Fox, I.; Specht, P. *J. Am. Mosq. Control Assoc.* **1988,** *4*, 163-167.
48. Gubler, D. J. *Am. J. Trop. Med. Hyg.* **1989,** *40*, 571-578.
49. Perich, M. J.; Davila, G.; Turner, A.; Garcia, A.; Nelson, M. *J. Med. Entomol.* **2000,** *37*, 541-546.
50. Spiegel, J.; Bennett, S.; Hattersley, L.; Hayden, M. H.; Kittayapong, P.; Nalim, S.; Wang, D. N. C.; Zielinski-Gutiérrez, E.; Gubler, D. *EcoHealth* **2005,** *2*, 273-290.
51. *Report of the Consultation on Key Issues in Dengue Vector Control, toward the Operationalization of a Global Strategy*; World Health Organization: Geneva, Switzerland, 2001.
52. Parks, W. J.; Lloyd, L. S.; Nathan, M. B.; Hosein, E.; Odugleh, A.; Clark, G. G.; Gubler, D. J.; Prasittisuk, C.; Palmer, K.; San Martin, J. L. *Dengue Bulletin* **2004,** *28*, 1-7.
53. Heintze, C.; Garrido, M. V.; Kroeger, A. *Trans. R. Soc. Trop. Med. Hyg.* **2007,** *101*, 317-325.
54. Gubler, D. J. *Clin. Microbiol. Rev.* **1998,** *11*, 480-496.
55. *State of the art of vaccine research and development.* WHO/IVB/05.XX; World Health Organization: Geneva, Switzerland, 2005.
56. Halstead, S. B.; Deen, J. *Lancet* **2002,** *360*, 1243-1245.
57. Almond, J.; Clemens, J.; Engers, H.; Halstead, S.; Khiem, H. B.; Pablos-Mendez, A.; Pervikov, Y.; Tram, T. T. *Vaccine* **2002,** *20*, 3043-3046.
58. Barrett, A. D.; Higgs, S. *Annu. Rev. Entomol.* **2007,** *52*, 209-229.
59. Farrar, J.; Focks, D.; Gubler, D.; Barrera, R.; Guzman, M. G.; Simmons, C.; Kalayanarooj, S.; Lum, L.; McCall, P. J.; Lloyd, L.; Horstick, O.; Dayal-

Drager, R.; Nathan, M. B.; Kroeger, A. *Trop. Med. Int. Health* **2007,** *12*, 695-699.
60. *Dengue and dengue hemorraghic fever in the Americas: guidelines for prevention and control*; Scientific Publication No. 548; Pan American Health Organization: Washington, DC, 1994.
61. *Report by the Secretariat: dengue prevention and control*; Provisional agenda item 13.14; World Health Organization: Geneva, Switzerland, 2002.
62. Morrison, A. C.; Zielinski-Gutierrez, E.; Scott, T. W.; Rosenberg, R. *PLoS Med.* **2008,** *5*, e68.
63. Lloyd, L. S. *Best Practices for dengue prevention and control in the Americas*; Strategic Report 7; Pan American Health Organization: Washington, DC, 2003.
64. Eisen, L.; Beaty, B. J. In *Vector-Borne Diseases: Understanding the Environmental, Human Health, and Ecological Connections*, Lemon, S. M.; Sparling, P. F.; Hamburg, M. A.; Relman, D. A.; Coffnes, E. R.; Mack, A., Eds. The National Academies Press: Washington, DC, 2008; pp 150-161.
65. Kuno, G. *Epidemiol. Rev.* **1995,** *17*, 321-335.
66. Tun-Lin, W.; Kay, B. H.; Barnes, A. *Am. J. Trop. Med. Hyg.* **1995,** *53*, 595-601.
67. Edman, J. D.; Scott, T. W.; Costero, A.; Morrison, A. C.; Harrington, L. C.; Clark, G. G. *J. Med. Entomol.* **1998,** *35*, 578-583.
68. Hemingway, J.; Beaty, B. J.; Rowland, M.; Scott, T. W.; Sharp, B. L. *Trends Parasitol.* **2006,** *22*, 308-312.
69. Getis, A.; Morrison, A. C.; Gray, K.; Scott, T. W. *Am. J. Trop. Med. Hyg.* **2003,** *69*, 494-505.
70. Knox, T. B.; Yen, N. T.; Nam, V. S.; Gatton, M. L.; Kay, B. H.; Ryan, P. A. *J. Med. Entomol.* **2007,** *44*, 192-204.
71. Romero-Vivas, C. M.; Falconar, A. K. *J. Am. Mosq. Control Assoc.* **2005,** *21*, 15-21.
72. Gubler, D.; Clark, G. C. *Emerg. Infect. Dis.* **1995,** *1*, 55-57.
73. Toledo, M. E.; Baly, A.; Vanlerberghe, V.; Rodriguez, M.; Benitez, J. R.; Duvergel, J.; Van der Stuyft, P. *Trop. Med. Int. Health* **2008,** *13*, 728-736.
74. Newton, E. A.; Reiter, P. *Am. J. Trop. Med. Hyg.* **1992,** *47*, 709-720.
75. Agudelo-Silva, F.; Spielman, A. *Am. J. Trop. Med. Hyg.* **1984,** *33*, 1267-1269.
76. Arrivillaga, J.; Barrera, R. *J. Vector Ecol.* **2004,** *29*, 11-20.
77. Igarashi, A. *FEMS Immunol. Med. Microbiol.* **1997,** *18*, 291-300.
78. Madarieta, S. K.; Salarda, A.; Benabaye, M. R. S.; Bacus, M. B.; Tagle Joseph, R., *Dengue Bulletin* **1999,** *23*, 51-54.
79. Nam, V. S.; Nguyen, H. T.; Tien, T. V.; Niem, T. S.; Hoa, N. T.; Thao, N. T.; Trong, T. Q.; Yen, N. T.; Ninh, T. U.; Self, L. S. *Dengue Newsletter* **1993,** *18*, 23-28.
80. Kroeger, A.; Lenhart, A.; Ochoa, M.; Villegas, E.; Levy, M.; Alexander, N.; McCall, P. J. *Brit. Med. J.* **2006,** *332*, 1247-1252.
81. Lenhart, A.; Orelus, N.; Maskill, R.; Alexander, N.; Streit, T.; McCall, P. J. *Trop. Med. Int. Health* **2008,** *13*, 56-67.
82. Mulla, M. S.; Tharvara, U.; Tawatsin, A.; Kong-Ngamsuk, A.; Chompoorsi, J. *J. Am. Mosq. Control Assoc.* **2001,** *17*, 153-159.

83. Hales, S.; van Panhuis, W. *Lancet* **2005,** *365*, 551-552.
84. Burkot, T.; Ichimori, K. *Trends Parasitol.* **2002,** *18*, 109-115.
85. Maxwell, C. A.; Mohammed, K.; Kisumku, U.; Curtis, C. F. *Bull. World Health Organ.* **1999,** *77*, 138-143.
86. Soper, F. L. *Am. J. Trop. Med. Hyg.* **1965,** *14*, 887-891.
87. Lardeux, F.; Riviere, F.; Sechan, Y.; Loncke, S. *Ann. Trop. Med. Parasitol.* **2002,** *96 Suppl 2*, S105-116.
88. *Strengthening implementation of the global strategy fro dengue fever/dengue haemorrhagic fever prevention and control: report of the Informal Consultation*; WHO/CDS/DEN(IC)/2000.1; World Health Organization: Geneva, Switzerland, 1999.
89. Sanchez, L.; Perez, D.; Perez, T.; Sosa, T.; Cruz, G.; Kouri, G.; Boelaert, M.; Van der Stuyft, P. *Trop. Med. Int. Health* **2005,** *10*, 82-91.
90. Nathan, M. B.; Knudsen, A. B. *J. Am. Mosq. Control Assoc.* **1991,** *7*, 400-404.
91. Rosenbaum, J.; Nathan, M. B.; Ragoonanansingh, R.; Rawlins, S.; Gayle, C.; Chadee, D. D.; Lloyd, L. S. *Am. J. Trop. Med. Hyg.* **1995,** *53*, 111-117.
92. Winch, P. J.; Leontsini, E.; Rigau-Perez, J. G.; Ruiz-Perez, M.; Clark, G. G.; Gubler, D. J. *Am. J. Trop. Med. Hyg.* **2002,** *67*, 363-370.

Chapter 5

Current Status and Challenges of Chagas Disease Control Initiatives in the Americas

Jun Nakagawa

Department of International Community Health, Graduate School of Medicine, University of Tokyo/ Japan International Cooperation Agency 2-2-15 Seko, Fujieda, Shizuoka, 426-0082, JAPAN

Chagas Disease Control Initiatives such as the Southern Cone Initiative and the Central American Initiative achieved reduction in the transmission of the disease via effective vector control. The Southern Cone Initiative triggered the launch of other regional initiatives such as the Central American, Andean and Amazon initiatives. The Central American Initiative made progress in the elimination of an imported triatomine (*Rhodnius prolixus*) and the control of a widespread native species (*Triatoma dimidiata*), while facing constraints such as a fragmented vector control program under a decentralized health system. International aid agencies and NGOs played an important role in Central America, in bridging between fragmented organizational resources. Decentralization of the health system limits the vertical vector control operation, and *T. dimidiata*-control needs sustainable surveillance and a control system to cover a large geographic area efficiently with stratification, quality control, community mobilization, and information management. Stakeholders such as the National Chagas Program, the local health system, and local government must share responsibilities to continue comprehensive vector control. Also, the private sector such as insecticide companies could be involved to explore alternative methods of spraying which complement the weakened institutional-led spraying, such as market- and incentive-driven spraying (purchase of insecticides and spraying by residents).

Introduction

Chagas disease is a parasitic infection in which the causative agent, a flagellate protozoan *Trypanosoma cruzi*, is transmitted to humans mainly through blood-sucking species of Triatominae, but also by blood transfusion, congenital transmission, and organ transplantation. Among these transmission pathways, vector-born transmission accounts for more than 80% of all transmission to humans (*1, 2*). *T. cruzi* is present in the feces of infected triatomine vectors, and enters the human body through bites, cuts or scratches on the skin and contact with mucous membranes.

The high economic impact of Chagas disease often severely affects the quality of life of those affected. WHO estimated that 16 to 18 million people were infected by *T. cruzi* (*3*). Although naturally present only in Latin America, Chagas disease is the fourth most serious parasitic disease in the world in terms of disability adjusted life years (DALYs) lost which is equivalent to over US$6.5 billion per year (*4*). The disease has a 5-15% mortality rate in the acute phase, especially amongst young children (*5*). Curative treatment of the infection is currently possible only during the acute and early chronic phase using one of two drugs – nifurtimox and benznidazole. Ten to 40% of infected individuals will develop severely debilitating lesions of organs such as the heart and digestive system (*5, 6*). The lack of vaccine and the difficulty in treatment makes vector control an important method for controlling Chagas disease transmission.

Success of the Attack Phase: "War" against Chagas disease

Elimination of transmission of Chagas disease is feasible, based on a well-established vector control strategy. The vector control program against triatomines significantly reduced Chagas disease transmission in South America. The incidence of Chagas disease was reduced from an estimated 700,000 cases per year to less than 60,000 (*6*). The Southern Cone Initiative (INCOSUR), was launched in 1991, to eliminate the main southern vector, *T. infestans*, and to eliminate transfusional transmission of *T. cruzi* in Argentine, Bolivia, Brazil, Chile, Paraguay, and Uruguay (*7*). The initiative successfully eliminated *T. infestans* over large areas of Uruguay, Chile, Brazil, Southern Argentine, and Western Paraguay, (see Figure 1) (*8, 9, 10*) This success suggested that Chagas disease control is no longer a technical issue, but a political and organizational issue (*11*).

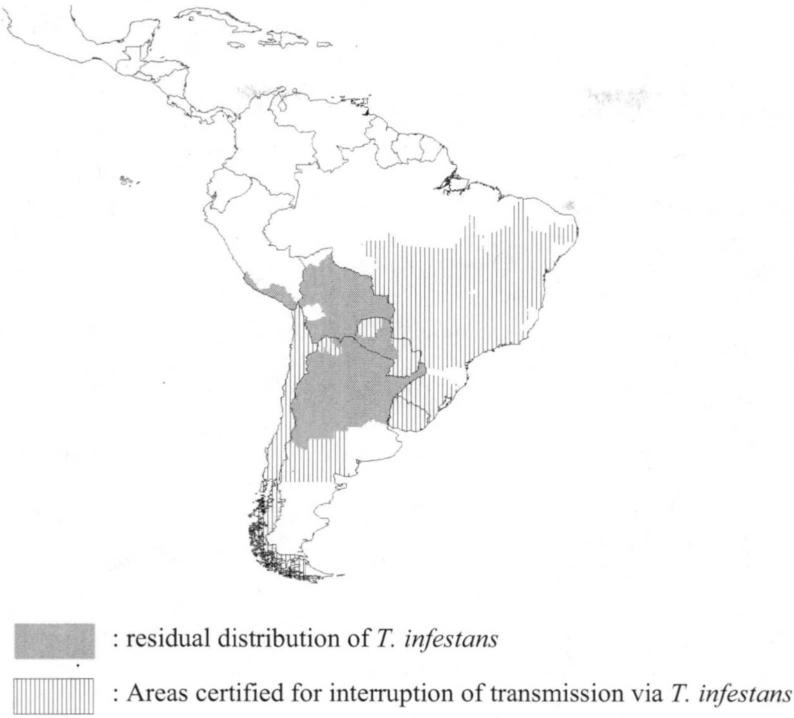

Figure 1. Current geographic distribution of *Triatoma infestans* (shaded). Area where interruption of Chagas disease transmission via *T. infestans* was certified, is shown in dots. Data from (*8*), (*9*), (*10*).

Vector control through indoor residual spraying of insecticides has been the most effective and economically efficient method for control. Domiciliated triatomines have biological characteristics different from other disease vectors such as mosquitoes, which function as key factors in facilitating their control: (a) relatively slow rate of repopulation development; (b) limited range of habitats, (c) limited dispersal during development; (d) susceptibility to modern pyrethroid insecticides with a low tendency to develop resistance, and (e) low genetic variability (*12*, *13*). Third-generation pyrethroids such as beta-cyfluthrin, (12.5% SC, at 25mg a.i./m^2), cyfluthrin (10% WP, at, 50mg a.i./m^2) deltamethrin (5% WP or 2.5% SC, at 25mg a.i./m^2) and lambda-cyhalothrin(10% WP, at 30mg a.i./m^2) proved to be highly effective for triatomine control (*14*, *15*).

Based on the success of the Southern Cone Initiative, the control of Chagas disease expanded to other regions such as Central America. The seven Central American countries, Belize, Costa Rica, El Salvador, Guatemala, Honduras, Nicaragua, and Panama, in 1997 launched the Central American Initiative (IPCA). Elimination of an introduced triatomine species, *R. prolixus*, and reduction of domestic infestation of a native species, *T. dimidiata*, has been the two main strategies to interrupt vector transmission of Chagas disease in Central

America. With its high natural infection rate and capacity to reach high densities, *R. prolixus* is a much more efficient vector than *T. dimidiata* in transmitting *T. cruzi* (*16*, *17*). The prevalence of human infection with *T. cruzi* is four times higher in villages infested with *R. prolixus* (38.8%) than in areas infested with *T. dimidiata* (8.9%) (*18*). *R. prolixus* is an exclusively domestic species in Central America, thus its elimination is feasible (*19*, *20*). Control of *T. dimidiata* is a challenge for Central America. *T. dimidiata*, a native species of Central America, has domestic, peri-domestic, and sylvatic populations, and cannot be eradicated from the region (*21*, *22*). Thus, the reduction of its intra-domestic population is the only feasible strategy against *T. dimidiata* and other native species (*23*, *24*).

The Central American Initiative drastically reduced the infestation level of *R. prolixus*, making its elimination feasible in the near future. Using the established vector control strategy, Guatemala, Nicaragua and Honduras, where *R. prolixus* was detected at the time of the launch of the regional initiative, applied insecticide spraying to all the infested villages. Guatemala, where most of the *R. prolixus*-infested villages existed, reduced the number of infested villages from 296 to 3 (*25*), and was certified for interruption of Chagas disease transmission via *R. prolixus* in 2008 (see Figure 2) (*26*, *27*).

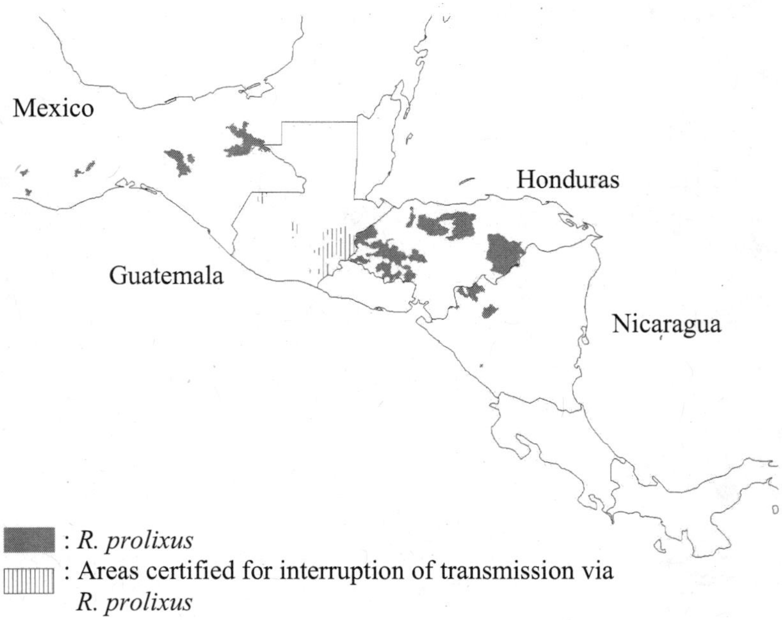

Figure 2. Current geographic distribution of *Rhodnius prolixus* in Central America and Mexico (black shaded). Area where interruption of Chagas disease transmission via *R. prolixus* was certified, is shown in dots. Data from (*25*), (*26*), (*27*).

Honduras sprayed 797 *R. prolixus*-infested villages, and Nicaragua identified 14 infested villages, and completed three cycles of insecticide spraying which should be sufficient to eliminate the species (*28*, *29*). Seroprevalence of children (7-15 years old) between 1998 and 2006 decreased in the most heavily infested municipalities in Guatemala from 12.1 to 4.5% in Jocotan, and from 11.6 to 1.6% in Camotan (*230*).

The control of *T. dimidiata* demonstrated reduction of its infestation level in Guatemala and El Salvador, though its re-infestation requires a sustainable and effective surveillance system. The Chagas disease control program in these two countries targeted insecticide spraying of villages with an infestation rate higher than 5%, and the entomological evaluation demonstrated the reduction of the infestation rate from 5.3% to 0.5% in Zacapa district, from 36.0% to 8.9% in Jutiapa district (*31*, *32*), and from 8.9% to 0.8% in Chalchuapa district in El Salvador (*33*). However, some apparent re-infestation was observed in areas with previously high infestation rates. Jutiapa health district in Guatemala reported re-infestation in 13 of 15 municipalities in the evaluation three years after the intervention (*34*).

This attack phase against *R. prolixus* and *T. dimidiata* overcame the challenges of executing effective vector control, with a well planned management strategy. The current issue for Chagas disease control is the maintenance of the integrity and quality of the national programs in the backdrop of a trend toward decentralization (*35*), which applies to Central America. When the Central American Initiative was launched in 1997, vertical organization and skilled personnel for vector control had almost disappeared from Central America. The attack phase against *R. prolixus* and *T. dimidiata* was organized with external assistance from organizations such as Japan International Cooperation Agency (JICA) which helped the national vector control program with technical assistance in logistics, resources and management (*36*). In a sense, the success of the vector control came from temporarily revitalizing the vertical vector control program.

Challenges: from "War" to "Peace-keeping"

Management of the vector control program, when the program phase enters the "maintenance phase", becomes an even greater challenge. The maintenance phase is long-term and requires sustainability, and a temporary fix is not a solution. When the risk is reduced, so is the cautious mindset. The major challenges for the maintenance of Chagas disease control is the maintenance of interest in Chagas disease control. After the certification of interruption of transmission of Chagas disease in Uruguay in 1998, for example, the government significantly reduced the budget for Chagas disease, which made sustainable surveillance of Chagas disease very difficult in Uruguay. When there is less visible risk, political interest declines, and that leads to insufficient resource allocation. The other challenge is the optimization of limited time and resources. The local health personnel are normally tied up with various activities such as immunization, and with vector control of other diseases such as dengue fever and malaria. Thus, integration of Chagas disease control as a routine activity, via efficient time and resource sharing with other activities, needs to be implemented. Maintaining a large geographic coverage of vector surveillance, in addition, is also a major challenge to sustain the low level of infestation. Existing entomological indices require trained vector personnel to conduct standard survey methods (such as the man-hour survey) and data analysis, which is sometimes too costly for the decentralized health administration.

The control of native species such as *T. dimidiata* requires an effective vector surveillance and control system which includes a) effective detection of re-infestation, b) stratification of high-risk areas and resource management, and c) response to the re-infestation (see Figure 3).

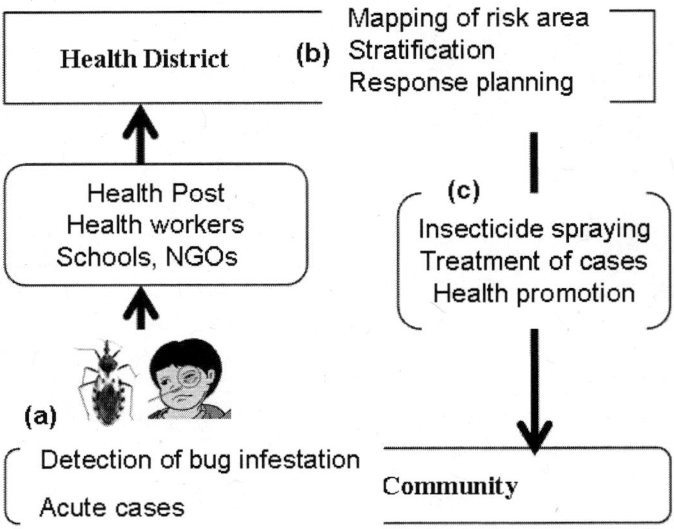

Figure 3. An example of the surveillance and control system of Chagas disease. The system includes three functions: (a) detection and reporting of bug infestation and acute cases; (b) stratification of high-risk areas and resource management, and; (c) response to the re-infestation.

The information on detection of bug infestation as well as any detection of acute disease cases should be reported to the closest health administration such as the Health Center. The local health administration office can detect high-risk areas based on the reporting, obtain necessary resources, and organize an institutional response to the reporting. Institutional responses include insecticide spraying, treatment of case patients, and educational activities. This vector surveillance and control system seems to work best when it is organized with community participation and at the administrative level closest to the community, to attain sufficient geographic coverage and to respond quickly to the bug re-infestation.

To establish an effective surveillance and control system for Chagas disease vectors with maximum quality and geographic coverage, the traditional vector control approach is not sufficient. We need to come up with an innovative approach.

Innovative Approach 1: Chagas Disease Campaign

Community-based campaign-style surveillance is an option for saving resources and time, although the data may not be as quantitative as the institutional survey. Organizing periodic triatomine-hunting campaigns to encourage residents to capture triatomines, can create a uniform hunting incentive to cover a large geographic area, and can obtain quantitative data such as the number of bugs captured per community, municipality, and department. Such data can be useful in making operational decisions and monitoring the level of infestation.

The campaign is a useful tool for public health activities, and is utilized for immunization, breast cancer, and HIV/AIDS. The campaign is normally a short-period, and its advantage is its resource mobilization, potential to cover large geographic areas, and visualization of activities. For Chagas disease control, a campaign can be organized for detection of bug-infestation and house-spraying.

A "Chagas week" was organized in August, 2007 in the municipality of San Pedro Pinula, Jalapa district in Guatemala to detect re-infestation of *R. prolixus*. In 2000, fifteen localities were infested with *R. prolixus*. After the two rounds of house spraying, no *R. prolixus* was reported since 2002, based on the surveillance activities by the vector control personnel of the district. The geographic coverage of the institutional surveillance, however, was limited due to a shortage of personnel. The campaign was aimed at obtaining a large geographic coverage of the surveillance in short period of time. The campaign period was set during the period when no other health-related activities were planed (to avoid coinciding with other activities such as dengue activities). Due to the short-period of the campaign, a large amount of resources was mobilized, such as vehicles not currently in use for immunizations and dengue control. Non-vector control personnel, schools, health centers, municipalities, and NGOs participated in the activity. During the campaign, triatomine collecting boxes were distributed to all 78 schools, combined with health promotion activities via radio, health centers, and health personnel, such as the vector control team, and community leaders. The campaign included attractive activities such as prizes (the student who captured *R. prolixus* or the most triatomines received a prize). 65.8% of schools reported infestation, among these, two localities were identified for *R. prolixus*-infestation (*37*).

This example demonstrated that the campaign method attained better geographic coverage in a short period of time, as well as better quality (by detecting *R. prolixus* which was not detected by the routine activities of the vector control personnel.) The campaign also attracted participation of children, schools, the municipality, NGOs, and the private sector.

Innovative Approach 2: Rapid Epidemiological Assessment

Another innovative strategy is "a school-based rapid epidemiological assessment" to stratify high-risk areas using a rapid serological test kit such as the Stat-Pak®. The traditional or vertical vector control program consists of a house-to-house entomological survey to stratify high-risk areas, and a vector control operation, which requires strong organizational capacity and resources. The rapid assessment strategy, initially proposed for *T. dimidiata*-control (*38*), sees the school as a catchment area for Chagas disease, deprioritizes the entomological survey, and focuses on disease detection and treatment and on recognition of the triatomine bug by students. In this strategy, in endemic areas, about 30 school children are randomly selected for the rapid serological test, and students are questioned about seeing the bug in their houses. The school catchment areas are then stratified based on seroprevalence, high risk (>10% seropositivity) and medium risk (3-10%). School catchment areas with no seropositivity and no recognition of the bug by students, are categorized as low risk (0%). High-risk areas are targeted for serological testing of the remaining school children, followed by quantitative ELISA for confirmation of positives, treatment of positive cases, as well as an entomological survey and insecticide spraying of all the positive houses. The medium-risk areas are targeted for confirmation of positive children via ELISA and treatment of all the positives, combined with an entomological survey and vector control. Then other schools in the surrounding areas will be targeted for the next rapid assessment.

This strategy optimizes time and resources. Focusing on case detection and bug recognition by students saves more time and resources than implementing an entomological survey. School-based serological surveys can grasp the epidemiological situation quickly, since schools are usually located in relatively accessible areas, and serological surveys can be performed efficiently with the presence of children from that area. Since triatomines have a relatively slow reproductive cycle with slow reinfestation, compared with other vectors such as mosquitoes, the rapid assessment can be implemented on a small scale, and the catchment areas can be gradually shifted to expand the geographic coverage over time. Honduras, one of the poorest countries in Latin America, adopted this strategy, and has reduced seroprevalence as well as house infestation level in the targeted communities (*28*).

Innovative Approach 3: Potential Partnership with Private Sector

The third innovation is to use incentives for residents and the private sector. In the Chagas disease endemic area, a large number of residents purchase rodenticides. Some residents have asked the vector control personnel about proper insecticides to spray against triatomines. The commonly applied products and spraying methods, however, are often not effective against triatomines. It is rare that the residents have the proper knowledge of products and basic spraying methods for effective triatomine control. If we can orient the residents to use the proper products and spraying methods as well as providing basic knowledge on Chagas disease, that can supplement the existing vector control activity via extending geographic coverage of the insecticide spraying. This may increase the incentive of the residents, the private sector, and the government via providing effective control methods for residents, creating a market for insecticide companies, and increasing coverage of vector control for the government. For example, the private sector can develop an informative package for insecticides, while the government and international organizations can provide educational materials which can be distributed via local agroservice stores. Or a health educational campaign to detect bug infestation and spraying can be organized as a partnership between public and private sectors.

This type of Public-Private Partnership (PPP) has good practices in the health sector, such as the epidemiological surveillance and control of iodine deficiency, which contributed to the improvement of health conditions (*39*). For example, the Central American Handwashing Initiative, a PPP among UNICEF, USAID, and private enterprises increased sales of soap, and resulted in an increase in the number of mothers who wash there hands with soap by 30% (*40*). These partnerships see the poor population as customers, a large market, and developed a successful business practice by creating profit for the enterprises as well as by meeting the needs of the poor to improve their living conditions. The same can be achieved for triatomine control, and may be engineered to improve the epidemiological surveillance of the disease. Opening distribution channels for the seller, for example, can contribute to vector surveillance by offering discounts for insecticides to buyers who bring triatomine bugs to the agroservice store. Records of purchases and locations of buyers can provide information on bug-reporting and house spraying which can be shared with the Ministry of Health.

While this PPP to increase the house-spraying activity is an attractive option, there are some issues that need to be resolved. Low effectiveness of residual spraying is normally observed when performed by untrained personnel. The standard sprayer for residual spraying, the Hudson spraypump, requires training and precise maintenance to perform effective residual spraying. The poorest population, in addition, is often affected most by Chagas disease, and can not afford to purchase necessary insecticides. Thus, house spraying by the Ministry of Health needs to be continued at least to cover the most affected areas as well as against triatomines targeted for elimination such as *R. prolixus* and *T. infestans*.

Conclusions

Based on the results of the regional initiatives, the elimination of Chagas disease transmission by 2010 is achievable in areas with imported species, such as *T. infestans* in Brazil, Chile, Southern Argentina, Uruguay, Eastern Paraguay, and *R. prolixus* in Guatemala and Northern Nicaragua. For sustainable control of Chagas disease under decentralized health systems, however, a combination of multiple strategies is the key.

Creation of political momentum is critical to tackle Chagas disease. The two recent political meetings, TICAD IV and the G8 summit in Japan emphasized the importance of Neglected Diseases control (*41*, *42*), which can provide an opportunity for an increase in resources. The recent establishment of the Neglected Disease Unit in the WHO and the launch of a new international initiative for sustainable elimination of Chagas disease transmission, which includes developed countries where cases were detected such as the U.S.A, Spain, and Japan (*43*), can play an important role to accelerate the effort. Institutionalization of vector-control activities, by optimizing the use of limited resources is also an approach. Innovative approaches can also increase the geographic coverage and sustainability of vector control. A Strategic Partnership with the private sector is also a key factor to do this. The recent agreement between WHO and Bayer on the donation of niflutimox (*44*) is a good example. A similar partnership can be achieved in Chagas disease vector control.

Acknowledgements

This article was written as part of the outcome of the Chagas disease control initiatives, and the author thanks Japan International Cooperation Agency, World Health Organization, Ministries of Health of Central and South American Countries, Medicins sans Frontieres and Canadian International Development Agency, and other organizations to their contribution for Chagas disease control. The work has benefitted from international collaboration through the ECLAT network, and the author also thanks Drs. C. Schofield, T. Hashimoto, H. Kawada, and C. Nakagawa, and Mr. K. Yoshioka for advice and collaboration to this article.

References

1. Dias, J.C. Chagas disease control in Brazil: which strategy after the attack phase? *Ann. Soc. Belg. Med. Trop.* **1991**, *71* (Suppl.1.), 75-86.
2. Marsden, P.D. The transmission of Trypanosoma cruzi infection to man and its control. In *Human Ecology and Infectious Disease*; Croll, N.A.; Cross, J.H., Ed.; Academic Press; New York, NY, 1983; pp 253-289.
3. WHO. *Control of Chagas Disease (Second Report)*; Technical Report Series No. 905; World Health Organization: Geneva, 2002, p109.
4. World Bank. *World Development Report 1993*; Oxford University Press: New York, NY, 1993, p329.
5. Schofield, C.J.; Dias, J.C. The Southern Cone Initiative against Chagas disease *Adv. Parasitol.* **1999,** *42*, 1-27.
6. Schofield, C.J.; Kabayo, J.P.; Trypanosomiasis vector control in Africa and Latin America *Parasit. Vectors*. **2008**, 1, 24.
7. WHO. *Control of Chagas Disease (Second Report)*. Technical Report Series No. 905; World Health Organization: Genera, 2002, p109.
8. PAHO. *Iniciativa del Cono Sur*; document no. PNSP/92-18. rev.1; Pan American Health Organization: Washington,D.C., 1993, p36.
9. PAHO. *XV^a Reunión de la Comisión Intergubernamental del Cono Sur para la Eliminación de Triatoma infestans y la Interrupción de la Transmisión de*

Tripanosomiasis Transfusional ; Pan American Heath Organization: Washington D.C.; http://www.paho.org/spanish/ad/dpc/cd/dch-incosur-xv.htm (accessed Jul 20, 2008).

10. PAHO. *XVII[a] Reunión de la Comisión Intergubernamental del Cono Sur para la Eliminación de Triatoma infestans y la Interrupción de la Transmisión de Tripanosomiasis Transfusional*, (in press).
11. Dias, J.C.; Silveira, A.C.; Schofield, C.J. The impact of Chagas disease control in Latin America: a review, *Mem. Inst. Oswaldo. Cruz.* **2002,** *97*, 603-612.
12. Dias, J. ; Schofield, J. The evolution of Chagas disease (American trypanosomiasis) control after 90 years since Carlos Chagas discovery, *Mem. Inst. Oswaldo. Cruz.* **1999,** *94*, Suppl 1: 103-21.
13. WHO. *Control of Chagas Disease (Second Report)*; Technical Report Series No. 905; World Health Organization: Geneva, 2002, p109.
14. Schofield, C. *Challenge of Chagas Disease Vector Control in Central America. Global Collaboration for Development of Pesticides for Public Health*; WHO/CDS/WHOPES/GCDPP/2000.1.; World Health Organization: Geneva, 2000, p36.
15. Zerba, E. *Past and Present of Chagas Vector Control and Future Needs, Global Collaboration for Development of Pesticides for Public Health*; WHO/CDS/WHOPES/GCDPP/99.1; Geneva: WHO, 1999, p14.
16. Ponce, C. Towards the elimination of the transmission of *Trypanosoma cruzi* in Honduras and Central American countries, *Medicina* (B Aires) **1999**, *59* Suppl 2, pp 117-119.
17. WHO. *Control of Chagas Disease (Second Report)*; Technical Report Series No. 905; World Health Organization: Geneva, 2002, p109.
18. Paz-Bailey, G.; Monroy, C.; Rodas, A.; Rosales, R.; Tabaru, R.; Davies, C.; Lines, J. Incidence of *Trypanosoma cruzi* infection in two Guatemalan communities, *Tran. R. Soc. Trop. Med. Hyg.* **2002**, *96*, 48-52.
19. Schofield, C. J.; Dujardin, J. P. Chagas disease vector control in Central America, *Parasitol. Today.* 1997, *13*, 141-144.
20. Dujardin, J. P.; Munoz, M.; Chavez, T.; Ponce, C.; Moreno, J.; Schofield, C. J. The origin of *Rhodnius prolixus* in Central America, *Med. Vet. Entomol.* **1998**, *12*, 113-115.
21. Acevedo, F.; Godoy, E.; Schofield, C. J. Comparison of intervention strategies for control of *Triatoma dimidiata* in Nicaragua, *Mem. Inst. Oswaldo. Cruz.* **2000**, *95*, 867-871.
22. Zeledón, R. *El Triatoma dimidiata (Latreille, 1811) y su Relación con la Enfermedad de Chagas*. Editora Universidad Estatal a Distancia: San José, Costa Rica; 1981, p146.
23. WHO. *Control of Chagas Disease (Second Report).* Technical Report Series No. 905. World Health Organization: Geneva, 2002, p109.
24. PAHO. *Iniciativa de Salud del Cono Sur. XIa. Reunión de la Comisión Intergubernamental para la Eliminación de* Triatoma infestans *y la Interrupción de la* Tripanosomiasis americana *por Transfusión*; document no. OPS/HCP/HCT/216/02; Pan American Health Organization: Washington, D.C: , 2002, p145.

25. Alvarez, H. *75 años del descubrimiento de la enfermedad de Chagas en Guatemala,* August 28, 2007, Presented at the 10th Annual Meeting of the Central American Initiative for Chagas Disease Control, Managua, Nicaragua, 2007.
26. PAHO, *Undécima reunión de la comisión intergubernamental de la iniciativa de los países de Centro América (IPCA) para la interrupción de la transmisión vectorial, transfusional y atención médica de la enfermedad de Chagas*, Washington, D.C: Pan American Health Organization (in press).
27. Campos, C. Distribución de los triatominos en México, in *Iniciativa para la vigilancia y el control de la enfermedad de Chagas en la República Mexicana*; Ramsey, J.; López, A.; Pohls, J. ,Eds; Instituto Nacional de Salud Pública; Cuernavaca, 2003, pp105-123.
28. Secretaría de Salud de Honduras; JICA. *Informe final Proyecto de Control de la Enfermedad de Chagas en Honduras 2003-2007*, Secretarial de Salud: Tegucigalpa, 2007, p50.
29. Marin, F., *Avances de Nicaragua Iniciativa Centroamericana IPCA (Nov. 1998 – Junio 2007)*, August 28, 2007, Presented at the 10th Annual Meeting of the Central American Initiative for Chagas Disease Control, Managua, Nicaragua, 2007.
30. Alvarez, H. *75 años del descubrimiento de la enfermedad de Chagas en Guatemala,* August 28, 2007, Presented at the 10th Annual Meeting of the Central American Initiative for Chagas Disease Control, Managua, Nicaragua, 2007.
31. Nakagawa, J.; Cordon-Rosales, C.; Juárez, J.; Itzep, C., Nonami, T. Impact of residual spraying on *Rhodnius prolixus* and *Triatoma dimidiata* in the district of Zacapa in Guatemala. *Mem. Inst. Oswaldo. Cruz.* **2003**, *98*, 277-81.
32. Nakagawa, J.; Hashimoto, K.; Cordon-Rosales, C.; Abraham Juárez, J.; Trampe, R.; Marroquín Marroquín, L. The impact of vector control on *Triatoma dimidiata* in the Guatemalan district of Jutiapa, *Ann. Trop. Med. Parasitol.* **2003**, *97*, 288-297.
33. Ramos, H.; Romero, E.; Serpas, *M., Situación epidemiológica de la Enfermedad de Chagas en El Salvador 2007*, March 27, 2008, presented at WHO-JICA-ECLAT meeting on the Designing of investigation on Chagas disease transmission levels by *Triatoma dimidiata*, a native vector of Central America, Geneva, 2008.
34. Trampe, R., personal communication, May 20, 2008.
35. Schofield, C.J.; Dias, J.C. The Southern Cone Initiative against Chagas disease, *Adv. Parasitol.* **1999**, *42*, 1-27.
36. Yamagata, Y.; Nakagawa, J. Control of Chagas disease, *Adv. Parasitol.* **2006**, *61*, 129-165.
37. Nakagawa, J.; Yoshioka, K., *Lecciones Aprendidas en el control de la enfermedad de Chagas en Centroamérica*, August 29, 2007, presented at the 10th Annual Meeting of the Central American Initiative for Chagas Disease Control, Managua, Nicaragua, 2007.
38. Schofield, C.; Jannin, J.; Salvatella, R., The future of Chagas disease control, *Trends. Parasitol.* **2006**, 22, 583-588.

39. Prahalad, C. *The Fortune at the Bottom of the Pyramid*; Wharton School Publishing: Upper Saddle River, NJ, 2005, p304.
40. The Global Public-Private Partnership to Promote Handwashing with Soap, http://www.globalhandwashing.org/Publications/Attachments/brochure.pdf, (accessed Jul 28, 2008).
41. TICAD IV Yokohama Action Plan, http://www.mofa.go.jp/region/africa/ticad/ticad4/doc/actoin.pdf, (accessed Jul 28, 2008).
42. Toyako Framework for Action on Global Health - Report of the G8 Health Experts Group - G8, http://www.g8summit.go.jp/doc/pdf/0708_09_en.pdf, (accessed Jul 28, 2008).
43. New global effort to eliminate Chagas disease, 2008, http://www.who.int/mediacentre/news/releases/2007/pr36/en/, (accessed Jul 28, 2008).
44. WHO expands fight against Chagas disease with support from Bayer, http://www.who.int/mediacentre/news/notes/2007/np16/en/, (accessed, Jul 28, 2008).

Chapter 6

Human Head Lice: Status, Control and Resistance

J. Marshall Clark[1], Si Hyeock Lee[2], Kyong Sup Yoon[1], Joseph P. Strycharz[1], and Deok Ho Kwon[2]

[1]Department of Veterinary & Animal Science, University of Massachusetts, Amherst, MA 01003
[2]Department of Agricultural Biotechnology, Seoul National University, Seoul, Korea 151-742

Pediculosis, caused by Pediculus lice, is the most prevalent parasitic infestation of humans. Most people find lice intolerable and repeatedly and prophylactically apply pediculicides. Commercial pediculicides are limited and health providers are spending an increasing amount of time and resources dealing with infestations. Few alternatives exist when standard treatments fail. U.S.pediculicide sales were last estimated at >$150 million just for over-the-counter (OTC) remedies and overall cost of infestations is ~ $1 billion annually. Infestation rates range from 6-12 million cases annually with 2.6 million households affected and 8% of all schoolchildren infested. Louse resistance to most commercial pediculicides is now commonly reported and increasing in frequency, particularly to DDT, pyrethrins, pyrethroids, and malathion. Knockdown resistance (kdr) is a major factor worldwide in all pyrethrin/pyrethroid-resistant lice studied to date. Recent genotyping efforts have determined that kdr resistance is widespread but not yet uniform. Malathion (e.g., Ovide®) is prescribed most often when pyrethroids fail. However, U.S. lice have widespread but low levels of malathion resistance. Enhanced malathion carboxylesterase activity is a major mechanism associated with highly malathion-resistant lice from the U.K.

The human head louse, *Pediculus humanus capitis* (L.), belongs to the hemimetabolous order Phthiraptera and is a blood-sucking, obligate ectoparasite of the human scalp. Although not a significant disease vector, head lice represent a major economic and social concern in North America and worldwide because infestations are often associated with school-aged children, who miss substantial school days (12-24 million days) during this critical learning period (*1*). Parents who must miss work to care for children who are sent home can also lose income. Infestations often cause intense itching, which can injure skin allowing secondary infections and self-inoculation of *Rickettsia prowazekii, Borrelia recurrentis,* and *Bartonella quintana* (*2*) and likely other bacteria such as Methicillin-resistant *Staphylococcus aureus* (MRSA).

Status of Pediculosis and Its Treatment

Pediculosis is the most prevalent parasitic infestation of humans (*3*). Acquired immunity likely reduces louse density and impact on chronically exposed older juveniles and adults. However, louse outbreaks may constitute one of many opportunistic infestations associated with a depressed immune system (e.g., people with HIV). Most people find lice intolerable and repeatedly and prophylactically apply pediculicides (insecticides) without realizing the harm and lethality if misused or overused. Misapplications affect children in particular due to their small size and higher sensitivity to the toxic effects of pediculicides (*4*).

There are two ways to combat pediculosis: 1) proactive prevention or 2) post-infestation treatment. Emphasis is increasingly on prevention (education) and physical removal (combing or shaving) because a crisis exists in the chemical management of pediculosis. The pediculicide arsenal is limited and shrinking due to decreasing efficacy and parents and health providers are spending an increasing and inordinate amount of time and resources dealing with infestations. Effective management information is generally lacking and few, if any, alternatives exist when standard treatments fail.

U.S. pediculicide sales are >$240 million per year with the over-the-counter (OTC) remedies accounting for > $90 million. Infestation rates range from 6-12 million cases annually with 2.6 million households affected and 8% of all school children infested (*5*). Overall cost of infestations is estimated at ~$1 billion annually but the long-term impact of days of lost learning by almost 1 in every 10 school-aged children due to the No-Nit policy and the lack of effective control options overshadows these cost estimates (*6*).

Commercial pediculicides that are currently in use consist of the OTC products and those available by prescription only (R_x) (Table I) (*7*). Currently, the OTC products comprise 70% of the pediculicides sold in the U.S. The OTC products consist of either pyrethroid insecticides (e.g., NIX®, 1% permethrin crème rinse, ~16% of the OTC market) or synergized pyrethrins (e.g., Rid®, Clear®, Pronto®, A-200®, ~0.3% with 3-4% piperonyl butoxide (PBO), an oxidative metabolic inhibitor, ~7-35% of the OTC market). The R_x market includes malathion (Ovide®, 0.5%, ~50% of the R_x market), lindane (Kwell®), permethrin (Elimite®), and ivermectin (IVOMEC®). Ovide® is prescribed most often when pyrethroids fail. Because of the dominance of the pyrethrins/pyrethroids and malathion in the current pediculicide market, the remainder of this chapter will focus on these insecticides.

Table I. Pediculicidal insecticides and products

Insecticide	Brands	Product Form	Dosage
OTC products			
Permethrin (1 %)	NIX	Crème Rinse	1 Application [a]
Pyrethrum (0.3-0.33 % with piperonyl butoxide 3-4 %)	RID, Clear, Pronto, A-200, various generics	Shampoo or Mousse	2 Applications, 7 -10 days apart
R_x products			
Malathion (0.5%)	Ovide	Alcoholic Lotion	1 Application
Lindane (1 %)	Various generics	Shampoo or Lotion	1 Application [a]
Permethrin (5 %)	Elimite	Cream	1 Application
Ivermectin (0.4 % w/v)	IVOMEC	Oral	1 Application

[a] A second application is required after 7 days if infestation persists.

Pyrethrins are natural apolar esters that are solvent-extracted from the flower heads of *Chrysanthemum cineraiaefolium.* They are excellent insecticides with low toxicity to mammals due to their poor absorption and rapid metabolism to non-toxic metabolites. Unfortunately, they are also rapidly broken down in the environment by photolysis and hydrolysis, making them unsuitable as field-applied insecticides. Permethrin, a synthetic pyrethrin called a pyrethroid, was designed as a field-stable insecticide by removing sites of photolytic degradation and xenobiotic metabolic attack. Both, along with DDT, share a common mode of action as agonists at voltage-gated sodium channels (VGSC) in the nervous systems of insects. Because of this, they both also share a common resistance mechanism with DDT, knockdown resistance (kdr), which is due to selective point mutations in the α-subunit of the VGSC that results in nerve insensitivity to these channel agonists.

Malathion is an organophosphorous insecticide (OP) of the phosphorodithioate subclass. It acts as an irreversible inhibitor of acetylcholinesterase within the synapse of cholinergic neurons. While most OP insecticides are extremely toxic to both insects and mammals, malathion is selectively toxic to insects because mammals carry out an enhanced hydrolysis of the carboxyl esters that are located in the alcohol moiety of this thiophosphoric acid esters. The resulting α- and β-malathion monoacids are too polar to bind acetylcholinesterase, making malathion one of the safest OP insecticides.

Resistance to Pyrethrins/Pyrethroids and Malathion

Pyrethrum (the natural pyrethrin extract) has been used to control ectoparasites, including lice on humans, since ancient times. Pyrethroids, including d-phenothrin and permethrin, have been registered as pediculicides since the 1970s and have been widely available as OTC products since the 1980s. Pediculicide treatment with malathion has been practiced for more that 80 years (*8*) and currently with Ovide®, a R_x product reintroduced in 1999. Despite these introductions of effective pediculicides, the number of cases of louse infestation has increased worldwide since the mid-1960s (*5*) and dramatically since the mid-1990s.

It has been long assumed that the loss of efficacious control is due, in part, to the development of insecticide resistance in head louse populations. As illustrated in Table II, this appears to be the case. Resistance to the pyrethroid pediculicides was first reported in France in 1994, followed by additional reports from other European countries (Czech Republic, UK, and Denmark), the Middle East (Israel), North (United States) and South (Argentina) America, Asia (Japan) and Australia. Currently, five of these countries have established that these pyrethroid products have failed clinically. There are studies now underway in Japan, EU and Canada to determine if clinical failure to the pyrethrin/permethrin OTC products has likewise occurred. Resistance to malathion has also been reported in head louse populations from France in 1995 (*9*), the United Kingdom in 1999 (*10*) and Australia in 2003 (*11*).

Unfortunately, much of the published work on the level of insecticide resistance in head lice and on the possible mechanisms involved is largely anecdotal and unreplicated. This problem stemmed from the lack of laboratory colonies of insecticide-susceptible and -resistant head lice necessary to standardize bioassay protocols. Over the past 5 years, a series of papers from the Clark research group describes the development of an *in vitro* rearing system for human head lice that has resolved this dilemma (*12,13,14*). The most current rendition of the *in vitro* rearing system is based on a silicone-reinforced Parafilm® M feeding membrane, human hair tufts and stirred, reconstituted human blood, assembled as diagramed in Figure 1. The *in vitro* rearing system, as configured, allows the large-scale rearing of head and body louse colonies. Each rearing vessel maintains 100-150 first or second instars and ~ 50 third instars or adults. This format allows ~1125-1800 eggs per day to be produced in the 15 rearing units on a single multipoint magnetic stirrer. The mean survivorship of three head louse strains on the *in vitro* system was not significantly different from that determined *in vivo* using human volunteers (*14*).

Table II. History of pyrethroid resistance in the human head louse *Pediculus humanus capitis*

Location	Reference Year	Pyrethroid	Clinical Failure
France	Chosidow *et al.,* 1994	d-Phenothrin	Yes
Czech Republic	Rupes *et al.,* 1995	Permethrin	Yes
Israel	Mumcuoglu *et al.,* 1995	Permethrin	Yes
Argentina	Picollo *et al.,* 1998	Permethrin	Yes
United Kingdom	Downs *et al.,* 1999	Permethrin	Yes
United States	Pollack *et al.,* 1999	Permethrin	No
Japan	Tomita *et al.*, 2003	d-Phenothrin	No
Australia	Hunter and Baker, 2003	Permethrin	No
Denmark	Kristensen, 2005	Permethrin	No

Eight strains of human lice have been reared on the *in vitro* rearing system (Table III). Three strains (PA-HL, EC-HL and IS-BL) have never been treated with pediculicides and serve as reference susceptible strains and five strains (BR-HL, CA-HL, FL-HL, MA-HL and TX-HL) have been previously treated with pediculicides. Median lethal time 50% values (LT_{50}) were determined for these strains using log time versus logit percent mortality regression analysis in conjunction with a contact bioassay based on insecticide-impregnated filter paper disks and resistance ratios (RR) calculated (*15*). As seen from the data presented in Table IV, permethrin resistance is widespread in the U.S. (MA, FL, TX, and CA) at a level of ~ 4-8 fold more than in the susceptible EC-HL strain. Additionally, the FL-HL and CA-HL strains show cross-resistance to pyrethrins and to PBO-synergized pyrethrins (~3 fold), and to DDT (~3 fold). These findings indicate that oxidative metabolism is not yet involved in pyrethrin/permethrin resistance in U.S. populations but target site insensitivity is likely.

Using a similar approach, resistance to malathion is also detected in the MA-HL, FL-HL and CA-HL strains at a level of 2-3 fold more than in the susceptible EC-HL strain. Malathion resistance is strongly synergized by the esterase inhibitor, DEF (Table IV, SF-HL), indicating that hydrolytic ester cleavage of malathion may be an important resistance mechanism.

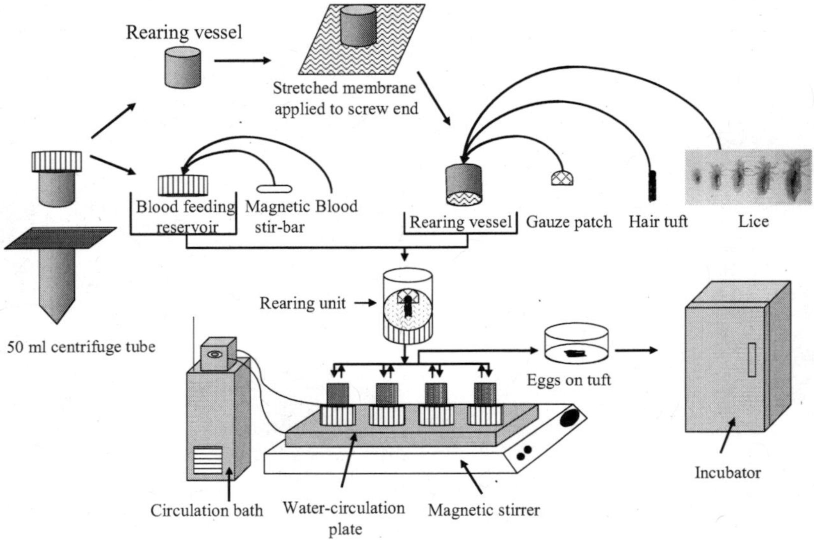

Figure 1. *Assembly of the in vitro rearing system.*
Reproduced with permission from reference 14. Copyright 2006 Elsevier.

In order to validate our initial resistance findings that were based on data derived from contact bioassays using only the insecticidal active ingredient, the *in vitro* rearing system was modified so that formulated pediculicide products could be assessed. Figure 2 illustrates the *Hair Tuft Mortality Bioassay*, which is based on applying formulated pediculicide products directly to a louse-infested human hair tuft following the manufacture's instructions (*14*). After treatment, the louse-infested hair tuft is placed back on the *in vitro* rearing system for assessment. This approach provides substantial improvements over existing bioassay formats for the assessment of head louse toxicity to pediculicides. First, lice are placed in an environment that simulates the human scalp in many ways and can feed and develop as normal. Because lice must feed every 10-12 hrs to survive, the lack of feeding in other bioassays artificially shortens the assessment interval to this time frame. Second, formulated materials can be applied as instructed by the respective manufacturer. Third, lice are provided refugia similar to that provided on the human scalp. Forth, lice can lay eggs on the hair tuft so that ovicidal activity (or the lack there of) can be assessed directly. The efficacies of three commercial pediculicidal products were assessed using the hair tuft bioassay in conjunction with the *in vitro* rearing system (Fig. 3). Treatments of 1% permethrin in acetone, Nix®, Rid®, or Pronto Plus® to hair tufts following manufactures' instructions were highly efficacious (100% mortality) on the susceptible EC-HL strain but differentially efficacious (62-84% mortality) on the permethrin-resistant strain from south Florida (SF-HL) when examined eight days post-treatment. SF-HL that survived the first treatment received an identical second treatment eight days following the first treatment. Survivors (13-30%) developed into adults, mated, and females laid fertile eggs that hatched into first instars. These results confirm resistance to permethrin- and pyrethrin-based pediculicidal formulations and validate resistance previously determined using filter-paper contact bioassays with unformulated neat insecticides.

Table III. Louse populations colonized on the *in vitro* rearing system.

Population	Source	Exposure to Pediculicides	Colonized
PA-HL	Niadup, Panama	No	Yes
EC-HL	Yamburara, Ecuador	No	Yes
IS-BL	Jeusalem, Israel	No	Yes
BR-HL	Bristol, United Kingdom	Yes	Yes
CA-HL	Los Angeles, CA	Yes	Yes
FL-HL	Plantation, FL	Yes	Yes
	Homestead, FL	Yes	Yes
MA-HL	Chicopee, MA	Yes	No
	Holyoke, MA	Yes	No
TX-HL	Corpus Christi, TX	Yes	No
	Mansfield, TX	Yes	No
	Mathis, TX	Yes	No
	San Antonio, TX	Yes	No

Table IV. Lethal time (LT_{50}, min) values and resistance ratios (RRs) from human head louse populations treated with currently-used pediculicides

Treatment	EC-HL LT_{50} (95% CL)	MA-HL LT_{50} (95% CL)	MA-HL RR[a]	SF-HL LT_{50} (95% CL)	SF-HL RR	TX-HL LT_{50} (95% CL)	TX-HL RR	CA-HL LT_{50} (95% CL)	CA-HL RR
1 % Permethrin	173 (121-237)	972 (938-1006)	5.6	1470 (1435-1505)	8.5	632 (591-673)	3.7	911 (855-963)	5.3
0.33 % Pyrethrum + 4 % PBO	508 (474-542)			1505 (1464-1548)	3.0			1296 (1257-1338)	2.6
10 % DDT	409 (368-451)			870 (822-917)	2.1			1379 (1326-1424)	3.4
0.5 % Malathion	122 (86-169)	290 (270-308)	2.4	239 (220-259)	2.0			398 (378-419)	3.3
0.5 % Malathion + 0.1 % DEF	111 (78-148)			91 (59-126)	0.8			399 (377-418)	3.6

[a] RR, mortality resistance ratio = LT_{50} (MA-HL, FL-HL, TX-HL or CA-HL)/LT_{50} (EC-HL).

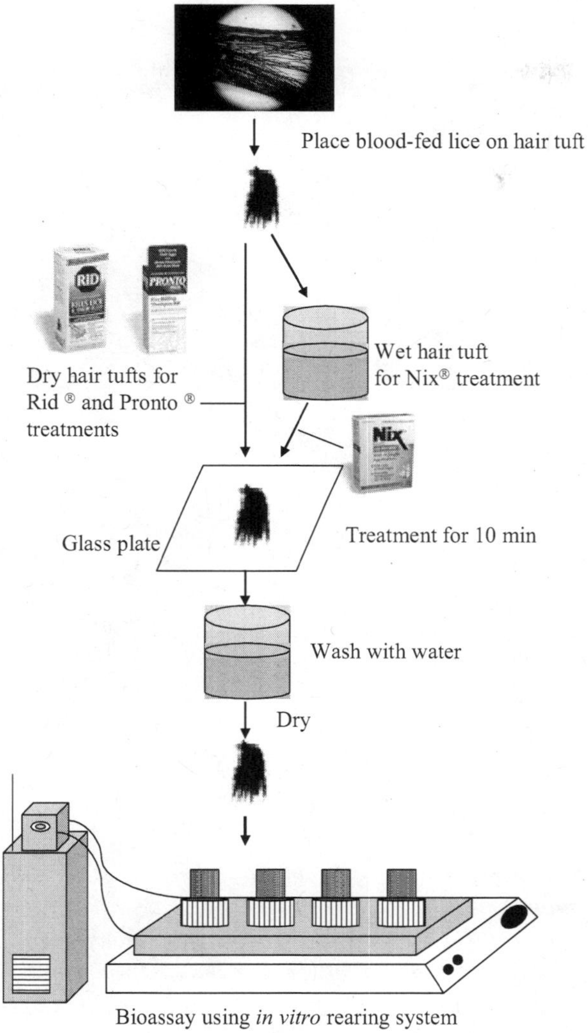

Figure 2. *The hair tuft mortality bioassay procedure performed on the in vitro rearing system to determine efficacy of pediculicidal products.* Reproduced with permission from reference 14. Copyright 2006 Elsevier.

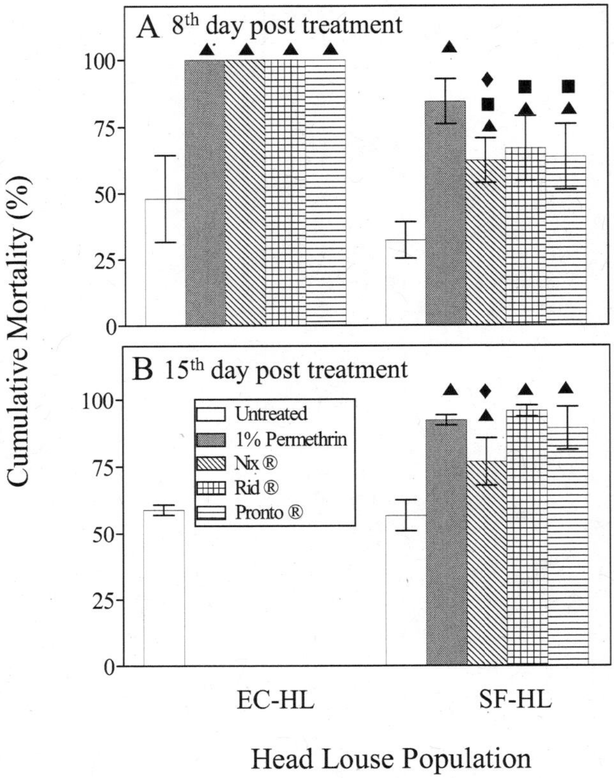

Figure 3. *Cumulative mortality of pediculicide-susceptible (EC-HL) and permethrin-resistant (SF-HL) head louse strains treated with 1 % permethrin in acetone, Nix®, Rid® or Pronto Plus® using the hair tuft bioassay in conjunction with the in vitro rearing system. Filled triangle (▲) indicates that treatment is significantly more efficacious compared to untreated lice of the same strain (t-test, p < 0.05). Filled square (■) indicates that SF-HL strain is more resistant to the treatment of OTC pediculicide compared to the respective treatments using the EC-HL strain (t-test, p < 0.05). Filled diamond (♦) indicates that the SF-HL strain is more resistant to Nix® treatment than to 1 % permethrin treatment.* Reproduced with permission from reference 14. Copyright 2006 Elsevier.

Resistance Mechanisms to Pediculicides

Mechanisms of Resistance to Permethrin

Lee *et al* (*16*) hypothesized that permethrin-resistant head lice most likely elicited a *knockdown resistance* (kdr) that arose from point mutations within the α-subunit gene of the voltage-gated sodium channel in the nervous system. Amino acid replacements decrease the affinity of the channel to permethrin, other pyrethroids, the pyrethrins, and DDT. Their conclusion was based on the fact that permethrin-resistant head lice were cross-resistant to DDT, only showed low levels of metabolic synergism, and were tolerant to knockdown in behavioral bioassays.

Molecular Analysis of kdr-type Resistance in Permethrin-Resistant Head Lice

Using a homology probing strategy, cDNA fragments that spanned the IIS4~IIS6 region of *para*-orthologous head louse sodium channel α-subunit gene, where most of the mutations associated with kdr are located, were PCR amplified (*16*). Through molecular cloning and sequencing, two point mutations, T929I and L932F (T917I and L920F in the numbering of the head louse amino acid sequence), located in the IIS5 transmembrane segment of cDNAs from only the permethrin-resistant FL-HL and BR-HL populations, were identified.

Sequence comparisons of the complete open reading frames of the sodium channel genes identified one additional novel mutation (M815I), which was located in the IIS1-2 extracellular loop of the α-subunit from only the permethrin-resistant head louse population (*17*). Sequence analyses of cloned cDNA fragments and genomic DNA fragments from individual louse samples, both containing the three mutation sites, confirmed that all the mutations exist *en bloc* as a resistant haplotype. Northern blot analysis identified a single 7.2 kb transcript.

Functional Significance of Louse Sodium Channel Mutations

The three louse mutations were inserted in all combinations using site-directed mutagenesis at the corresponding amino acid sequence positions (M827I, T929I and L932F) of the house fly *para*-orthologous voltage-sensitive sodium channel α-subunit ($Vssc1^{WT}$) gene and heterologously co-expressed with the sodium channel auxiliary subunit of house fly (Vsscβ) in *Xenopus* oocytes (*18*). The M827I and L932F mutations reduced permethrin sensitivity when expressed alone but the T929I mutation, either alone or in combination, virtually abolished permethrin sensitivity (Fig. 4). Thus, the T929I mutation is the principal cause of permethrin resistance in head lice via a kdr-type nerve insensitivity mechanism.

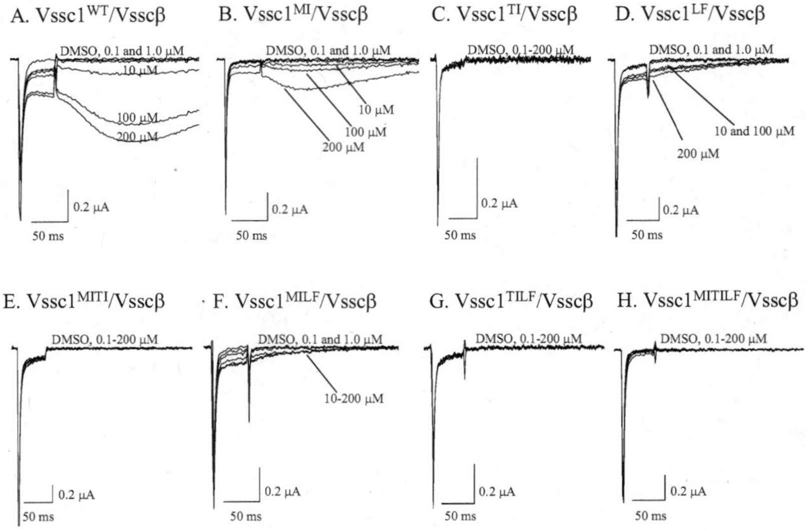

Figure 4. *Comparative sodium current traces from Xenopus oocytes obtained before and after exposure to increasing concentrations of permethrin.* Reproduced with permission from reference 18. Copyright 2008 Elsevier.

Mechanisms of Resistance to Malathion

Malathion resistance was first reported from the United Kingdom in two head louse populations that were also resistant to permethrin (10). Low levels of malathion resistance was recently reported in head louse populations from Florida and southern California (*15*), which suggests that malathion resistance is likely to expand with the increased use of malathion-containing products. Yoon *et al* (*15*) first hypothesized that enhanced hydrolytic xenobiotic metabolism (e.g., malathion carboxylesterase) was like involved due to high levels of DEF synergism seen in both the permethrin/malathion resistant strain from the United Kingdom (BR-HL) and in the south Florida population (SF-HL).

Increased Carboxylesterase Activity and Formation of Malathion Monoacids
Non-denaturation (native) PAGE analysis of the 15,000g supernatant of malathion-susceptible (EC-HL) and -resistant (BR-HL) head lice treated with α-naphthyl acetate and stained with Fast Garnet GBC dye is presented in Figure 5 (*19*). Two prominent bands (E1 and E3) are increased in the BR-HL supernatant and an additional band (E2) with high activity appears only in the BR-HL supernatant (Fig. 5, left side). Densitometric analysis of the gel revealed that E1 activity of the BR-HL strain was increased 6-fold over that of the EC-HL strain and E3 by 2-fold (Fig. 5, right side). Malathion (^{14}C-lableled) and its carboxylesterase-generated metabolites (α- and β-monoacids) were well separated and quantified by TLC-radiometric analysis (Fig. 6). The amount of malathion was significantly less in the BR-HL lanes compared to the EC-HL lanes, whereas the later was not significantly different from that detected in the

control lanes. The amount of malathion monoacids was significantly higher in the BR-HL lanes than that in the EC-HL lanes, whereas the later was not significantly different from that detected in the control lanes. The carboxylesterase inhibitor, TPP, reduced the conversion of malathion to its monoacids to a level that was not significantly different from that obtained from the EC-HL preparation. Based on these amounts, the BR-HL strain had ~13-fold higher malathion carboxylesterase activity compared with EC-HL lice.

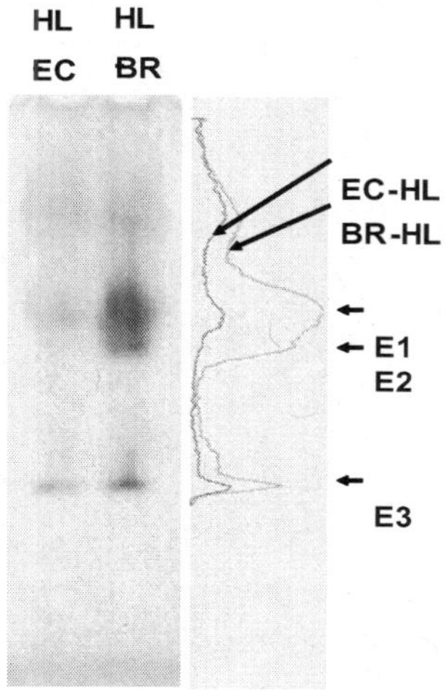

Figure 5. Polyacrylamide gel electrophoresis of esterases from human head lice (left panels) and densitograms (right panel). Reproduced with permission from reference 19. Copyright 2006 Elsevier.

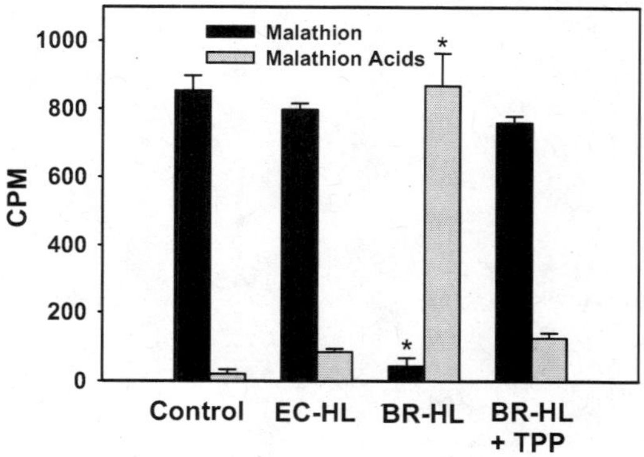

Figure 6. In vitro degradation of [2,3-^{14}C]malathion head lice adults as determined by TLC. Means (counts per minute, CPM, ± SD) with asterisks are significantly different compared to control or EC-HL values (Duncan's multiple range test, P<0.05).Reproduced with permission from reference 19. Copyright 2006 Elsevier.

Quantitative real-time PCR (qPCR) of malathion carboxylesterase gene in malathion-resistant BR-HL lice

PhumU1.1 peptide database (http://phumanus.vectorbase.org/Tools/Blast/) was searched by Blastp and six carboxylesterases (HLCbE1-6) identified. Total RNA was extracted from 35 female lice of the susceptible PA-HL strain or the malathion-resistant BR-HL strain. Generation of cDNAs and qPCR were carried out using standard protocols (*20*). Among the 6 putative carboxylesterases (HLCbE1-6), a single gene (PHUM005138) was significantly over-transcribed in the BR-HL compared to the PA-HL lice (5.4-fold), indicating the HLCbE4 is the most likely candidate as the malathion carboxylesterase responsible for malathion metabolism and resistance (Table V).

Table V. Transcription levels of HLCbEs in the insecticide-susceptible PA-HL and malathion-resistant BR-HL strains of human head lice

CbE	Transcript ratio (CbE/Actin)		Ratio (BR/PA)	p-value
	PA-HL	BR-HL		
HLCbE1 (PHUM000301)	0.37 ± 0.03	0.247 ± 0.02	0.66	0.007
HLCbE2 (PHUM005821)	0.053 ± 0.005	0.021 ± 0.006	0.39	0.0018
HLCbE3 (PHUM010024)	0.013 ± 0.001	0.016 ± 0.004	1.24	0.299
HLCbE4 (PHUM005138)	0.09 ± 0.25	0.499 ± 0.132	5.4	0.0009
HLCbE5 (PHUM006997)	0.032 ± 0. 006	0.027 ± 0.002	0.80	0.31
HLCbE6 (PHUM001288)	0.002 ± 0.0003	0.001 ± 0.0003	0.5	0.036

Conclusions

Permethrin resistance has been reported worldwide and clinical failures of commercial pediculicides containing permethrin have likewise occurred. Permethrin resistance in head lice populations from the U.S. is widespread but is not yet uniform and the level of resistance is relatively low (~4-8 fold). Permethrin-resistant lice are cross-resistant to pyrethrins, PBO-synergized pyrethrins and to DDT. Nix®, when applied to human hair tufts following manufacture's instructions, did not provide 100% control when assessed by the hair tuft bioassay in conjunction with the *in vitro* rearing system. Resistance to permethrin is due to knockdown resistance, which is the result of three point mutations within the α-subunit gene of the voltage-gated sodium channel that produces amino acid substitutions, leading to nerve insensitivity.

Malathion resistance has likewise been detected globally (France, the United Kingdom, Australia) and more recently low levels of malathion resistance has been detected in head louse populations from Massachusetts, Florida and California. High levels of DEF synergism and increased levels of carboxylesterase activity in malathion-resistant lice (BR-HL) indicated that malathion carboxylesterase was a likely mechanism. Enhance formation of monoacids from malathion by the malathion-resistant BR-HL strain validated this mechanism. Over-expression of a single carboxylesterase gene (PHUM005138) from the BR-HL strain strongly suggests that HLCbE4 functions as a malathion carboxylesterase and is the cause of malathion resistance in this strain.

Need for New Pediculicides and Resistance Management

Insecticide resistance threatens the success of all vector control programs but is particularly problematic in the control of human lice for several reasons: 1) they are obligate human blood feeders that are exposed to pediculicides at all stages because most infestations are treated (few if any refugia); 2) they have low mobility, short generational time, and high fecundity; 3) there is a small and dwindling number of effective commercial pediculicidal products, the majority of which share common chemistry and elicit cross-resistance. These aspects combine and produce a *worst-case scenario* for the evolution of resistance in human lice.

Louse resistance to most commercial pediculicides has occurred and is increasing, particularly to DDT, pyrethrins, pyrethroids, and malathion. Current control and resistance problems underscore the need to understand the molecular mechanisms of insecticide resistance in human lice. For example, the genome sequence for *P. humanus humanus* has allowed the development of oligoarrays and the identification of a more complete complement of genes differentially expressed in pesticide-resistant strains (see Pittendrigh *et al,* this volume). The identification of such resistance mechanisms and novel target sites may allow the development of resistance-breaking compounds (e.g., negative cross-resistance compounds), DNA-based diagnostics for management (see Lee *et al,* this volume) and specific non-toxic synergists useful in novel strategies to control pediculicide-resistant populations.

Acknowledgements

This work was supported by the NIH/NIAID (R01 AI045062-04A3). S.H. Lee and D.H.Kwon were supported in part by the Brain Korea 21 Program.

References

1. Williams, L.K.; Reichart, A.; MacKenzie, W.R.; Hightower, A.W.; Blake, P.A. *Pediatrics.* **2001**, *107,* 1011-1015.
2. Jones, D.S.; Wache, S.; Chhokar, V. *Toxicon.* **1996,** *34*, 1421-1429.
3. Raoult, D,; Roux, V. *Clin. Infect. Dis.* **1999**, *29,* 888-911.
4. *Pesticides in the Diet of Infants and Children.* National Research Council. National Academies Press, Washington, D.C. 1993; pp 267-322.
5. Gratz, N.G. *Human Lice: Their Prevalaence, Control and Resistance to Insecticides.* WHO/CTD/WHOPES/97.8. World Health Org. Switzerland. 1997; pp. 61.
6. Barclay, L.; Vega, C. *Pediatrics.* **2007,** *119,* 965-975.

7. Bartels, C.L.; Peterson, K.E.; Taylor, K.L. *The Ann. Pharmacother.* **2001,** *35,* 109-112.
8. Auden, G.A. *Lancet.* **1921**, *198,* 370-375.
9. Izri, M.A.; Briere, C. *La Presse Medicale.* **1995,** *24*, 1444.
10. Downs, A.M.R.; Stafford, K.A.; Harvey, I.; Coles, G.C. *Br. J. Dermatol.* **1999**, *141,* 508-511.
11. Hunter, J.A.; Barker, S.C. *Parasitol. Res.* **2003**, *90*, 476-478.
12. Takano-Lee, M.; Yoon, K.-S.; Edman, J. D.; Mullens, B. A.; Clark, J. M. *J. Med. Entomol.* **2003,** *40*, 628-635.
13. Takano-Lee, M.; Velten, R.K.; Edman, J. D.; Mullens, B. A.; Clark, J. M. *J. Med. Entomol.* **2003**. *40*, 795-799.
14. Yoon, K.S.; Strycharz, J.P.; Gao, J.R.; Takano-Lee, M.; Edman, J.D.; Clark, J.M. *Pestic. Biochem. Physiol.* **2006,** *86*: 195-202.
15. Yoon, K.S.; Gao, J.-R.; Lee, S.H.; Coles, G.G.; Meinking, T.L.; Taplin, D.; Edman, J.D.; Takano-Lee, M.; and Clark, J.M. *Pestic. Biochem. Physiol.* 2004, *80*, 192-201.
16. Lee, S.H.; Yoon, K.S.; Williamson, M.S.; Goodson, S.J.; Takano-Lee, M.; Edman, J.D.; Devonshire, A.L.; and Clark, J.M. *Pestic. Biochem. Physiol.* **2000,** *66*, 130-143.
17. Lee, S.H.; Gao, J.-R.; Yoon, K.S.; Mumcuoglu, K.Y.; Taplin, D.; Edman, J.D.; Takano-Lee, M.; and Clark, J.M. *Pestic. Biochem Physiol.* 2003, *75*, 79-91.
18. Yoon, K.S.; Symington, S.B.; Lee, S.-H.; Soderlund, D.M.; Clark, J.M. *Insect. Biochem. & Mol. Biol.* **2008**, *38,* 296-306.
19. Gao, J.-R.; Yoon, K.S.; Frisbie, R.K.; Coles, G.C.; Clark, J.M. *Pestic. Biochem. Physiol.* **2006,** *85*, 28-37.
20. Kwon, D.H.; Clark, J.M.; Lee, S.H. 2004. *Pestic. Biochem. Physiol.* 2004, *78*, 39-48.

Chapter 7

The ABC's of Indoor Health:

Allergens, Baits, and Cockroach Mitigation Strategies

Coby Schal

Department of Entomology and W. M. Keck Center for Behavioral Biology, North Carolina State University, Raleigh, NC 27695-7613

The German cockroach, *Blattella germanica*, is a major structural pest, and cockroach allergens have been linked to the development and exacerbation of allergic disease and asthma in cockroach sensitive individuals. The inner-city residential environment often supports large cockroach infestations, which expose residents to high levels of allergens. This review summarizes information on the public health and veterinary importance of the German cockroach. It then presents a brief overview of the current status of various pest control options, with particular emphasis on insecticide baits and the role of horizontal transfer of active ingredient among cockroaches. Finally, I summarize experimental efforts to both eradicate cockroach infestations and to reduce allergen levels. Field studies show that intensive, targeted cockroach control with reduced-risk gel baits can lead to both dramatic reductions in cockroaches and clinically significant declines in cockroach allergens.

Human population growth and industrial development continue to lead to urbanization, especially in developing countries, where people move in large numbers from rural provinces to urban centers. The resulting urban mix of densely packed and crowded residences, centralized large-scale food processing and distribution, and a network of plumbing and sewer lines provides several commensal indoor pests easy access to, and dispersal within, the human-built environment.

While most indoor pests, including ants, bed bugs, beetles, fleas, flies, and termites are facultative commensals with humans, the German cockroach, *Blattella germanica*, stands alone as the only indoor pest with an obligate relationship with humans and human-built structures. A handful of the approximately 4,000 described cockroach species are considered pests – including *Supella longipalpa* (brownbanded), *Periplaneta americana* (American), *Periplaneta fuliginosa* (smokybrown), *Periplaneta australasiae* (Australian or Australasian), *Periplaneta brunea* (brown), *Blatta orientalis* (oriental), and *Eurycotis floridana* (Florida) – but the German cockroach remains the most important and is becoming so in more developing countries as indoor temperature and humidity are more ubiquitously managed in residential and other structural environments.

The German Cockroach: Public Health and Veterinary Pest

The German cockroach poses both direct and indirect hazards to humans and animals. The major reasons for suppressing indoor cockroach infestations and the choice of control options include public health, veterinary and aesthetic concerns, the harmful effects of insecticides to humans, pets and the environment, and regulatory requirements.

Cockroaches as Producers of Allergens

The prevalence and severity of asthma have been increasing dramatically over the past 40 years (*1*), and in the United States, asthma affects approximately 30 million people, 9 million of whom are children under the age of 18 (*2*); it is one of the most costly diseases, estimated at $12.7 billion annually (*3*). Although triggers of allergies and asthma are multifactorial, it is thought that the same changes in housing design that support cockroach infestations, as well as changes in human behavior (e.g., more time spent indoors) have resulted in prolonged human exposure to indoor aeroallergens of biological origins, including from cockroaches.

Because cockroach infestations can reach extremely high levels in homes and in industrial and agricultural situations (Figure 1), they pose risks from inhalant allergens. Approximately 26% of the U.S. population, aged 6 to 59, is sensitive to German cockroach allergens (*4*), and evidence suggests that exposure to cockroach allergen might be the most important risk factor for asthma in inner-city households. The National Cooperative Inner-City Asthma Study (NCICAS) found that asthma morbidity was highest in children with *both* a positive skin-test response and a high exposure to the cockroach allergen (*5*). Detectable levels of this cockroach allergen were found in 85% of the bedrooms tested, and 50% of the bedrooms had levels above the proposed threshold for allergic sensitization. The same study showed that 37% of inner-city children were allergic to cockroaches because of chronic exposure to cockroaches (*5*). Of the ~400,000 yearly emergency room admissions of adults with asthma, ~200,000 are associated with mite, cat, or cockroach allergens (*6*). In the NCICAS, children that were sensitive to cockroach allergens had a 3.4-times higher rate of hospitalization than other study cohorts, they made 78% more asthma-related unscheduled visits to health care providers, awoke more nights, and missed more school days (*5*). Other studies (e.g., *7*) have confirmed that cockroach allergen level is a good predictor of repeated wheezing and asthma. These measures of morbidity due to asthma highlight the medical and economic costs of cockroach infestations to society.

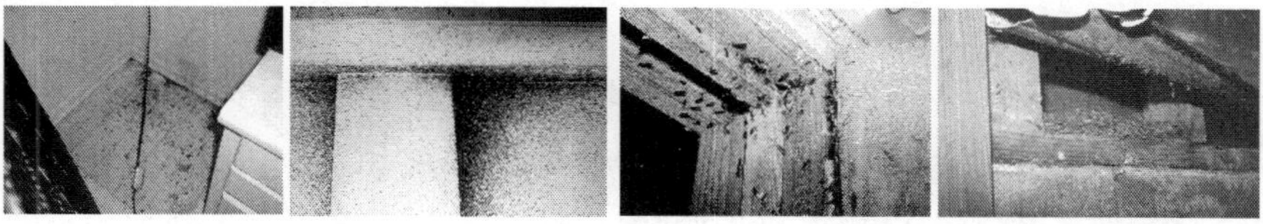

Figure 1. *Left to right: Cockroaches and cockroach "frass" behind the refrigerator of a cockroach-infested apartment; fecal smears on a wall in a cockroach-infested apartment (smears are laden with allergens); doorway of an infested pig farm in Eastern NC; and the wall void of an infested pig farm showing the large accumulation of cockroach feces and allergens.*

Cockroaches as Vectors of Pathogens and Antibiotic Resistant Microbes

Because cockroaches move freely between waste and food, they can acquire, carry, and transfer pathogenic bacteria, helminthes, fungi, protozoa, and viruses either mechanically or in their digestive system (*8*). A number of studies have implicated cockroaches as potential mechanical vectors of microbial pathogens to humans and animals (e.g., *9*, *10*). We recently screened the gastrointestinal microbial community of German cockroaches from several swine farms for antibiotic sensitivity in two clinically important bacterial species (Aqeel et al., unpublished). All isolates of *Enterococcus faecalis* and *Escherichia coli* were highly resistant to tetracycline. In addition, a high percentage of *E. faecalis* was also resistant to neomycin, erythromycin, chloramphenicol and vancomycin. *Escherichia coli* isolates were found to be resistant to streptomycin and cephalothin, two widely used antibiotics in medicine. In contrast, bacterial isolates from cockroaches collected in residences in Raleigh, North Carolina, exhibited only minor tolerance to tetracycline. Since cockroaches readily spread within the residential community, they could play a significant role in the epidemiology of antibiotic resistant strains.

We also examined the vector competence of German cockroaches for one of the most important bacterial pathogens of piglets, a verotoxigenic *Escherichia coli*. While most *E. coli* are non-pathogenic, several strains (containing specific virulence factors: toxins and pili/fimbriae) cause severe and sometimes life-threatening diarrhea, septicemia, or enterotoxemia in neonatal, young, and postweaning piglets as well as adult pigs (*11*). Using multiplex PCR for screening 4 virulence factors associated with this bacterial strain, we showed that this pathogen remained viable and virulent in the cockroach gut and feces for >8 days after the initial exposure (*12*). These preliminary results strongly implicate cockroaches in the mechanical dissemination of antibiotic resistant pathogenic microbes from places where they evolve antibiotic resistance (e.g., farms) to residential settings and potentially even to food processing.

Indirect Effects Related to Insecticide Use

Cockroaches are generally controlled with broad-spectrum neurotoxic insecticides. Insecticide use targeting cockroaches is widespread in inner-city communities, resulting in extensive indoor exposures to pesticides (*13*). Recent studies in New York City reported that 72% of recent mothers reported indoor insecticide exposure during pregnancy, and urine samples collected during delivery showed that 55% had detectable levels of a metabolite of the organophosphate chlorpyrifos, and 37% had detectable levels of a metabolite of pyrethroid insecticides (*14*). Another study in New York showed that 100% of participants had detectable airborne exposures to organophosphate and carbamate insecticides and these insecticides were detected in up to 74% of blood samples collected from mothers and newborns at delivery, implicating placental transfer of these compounds (*13*). There are several more such studies, all indicating that neurotoxic insecticides might have detrimental effects in the indoor environment (see *15*), including a recent examination of the relationship between household exposure to pesticides and the risk of childhood hematopoietic malignancies (*16*).

On average, >100 kg of active ingredient are applied annually on each swine farm to control cockroaches (Schal, pers. obs.). Most commonly, the least expensive, older pyrethroid insecticides are used in the U.S., and organophosphate and carbamate insecticides are used in other countries. Few of the newest insecticides and the modern baits are labeled for use around livestock. Although the older insecticides can effectively reduce cockroach populations if properly applied (*17*), they also expose people and animals to unnecessary health and environmental risks (review: *18*). Moreover, their efficacy becomes limited because insecticide resistance can develop rapidly in cockroach populations.

Economic Damage

Cockroaches tend to aggregate within electrical conduits, relays, and electronic switching equipment. There are no estimates of the cost of mechanical damage caused by cockroaches, but a conservative estimate of $1,000–$2,000 of damaged equipment per swine farm per year, not including interruption of production (feed not getting to hogs, warmers not working, sprinklers disrupted), and assuming a 30% infestation rate of large farms (based on an NCSU Extension survey), this impact alone amounts to $8.14 million in North Carolina alone. Unfortunately, there are no reliable estimates of the monetary cost of cockroach infestations in loss of contaminated food, restaurant closings, litigation, and loss of return customers (as for example, on cruise ships).

In light of the significant and harmful effects of cockroach infestations in residential settings, hospitals, farm structures, food-processing facilities and food warehouses, as well as in transportation networks and recreational settings, it is astonishing that aesthetic injury level (AIL) has become a widely adopted concept in urban entomology. While the occasional smokybrown or wood cockroach that is trapped in a home may pose aesthetic concerns to residents, German cockroach infestations in hospitals, nursing homes, and inner-city apartments clearly pose public health concerns – AIL applied to German cockroaches trivializes their public health importance.

Status of German Cockroach Control

Various approaches for controlling German cockroach infestations have been reviewed. Of particular interest are the following reviews: *18*, *19*, and *20*.

Habitat Modification, Physical Changes, and Mass Removal

Physical modification of the environment aims to reduce resources that sustain population growth, it stimulates movement to facilitate contact with residual insecticides, and it reduces the areas that require insecticide treatment. Structural modifications include maintenance of proper construction and sanitation, use of repellent sorptive dusts in wall and cabinet voids, sealing and caulking runways such as plumbing and electrical conduits between structures, removing resources such as food, water, and favorable shelters, treatment of structures with heat or freezing temperatures, and use of repellents to create "pest exclusion zones." Mass removal of cockroaches can be implemented with food- or pheromone-baited traps and vacuum devices. All these approaches, however, appear to be effective only in combination with efficacious formulations of insecticides. Gold (*21*) reviews alternative, non-pesticide-based approaches.

Biological Control Approaches

Although alternative approaches for cockroach control are sorely needed and it is essential that safe, effective, and environmentally compatible insect control techniques be developed and incorporated into sustainable IPM programs, biological control approaches are poorly developed for cockroaches (*22*, *23*). Parasitoids have been used with some success to reduce outdoor and greenhouse populations of the American, oriental, and brownbanded cockroaches. However, there are no known parasitoids of *B. germanica* and various parasitic nematodes, viruses, fungi, bacteria, and protozoa have been tested against the German cockroach, with generally unimpressive results (*23*).

Nevertheless, Zurek et al. (*17*) showed that concurrent dosing of German cockroaches with the fungus *Metarhizium anisopliae* and boric acid (either topically applied as a dust or diluted in drinking water) killed more cockroaches faster than either material alone. The synergistic interaction between these two insecticides needs to be explored in the field.

In the course of molecular ecology studies of cockroach populations, we recently discovered a new entomopathogenic densovirus, *Blattella germanica* DNV (*Bg*DNV). Infected cockroaches display several symptoms of pathology, including lethargy, flaccidity, poorly coordinated movements, and partial or complete paralysis of the hind legs (*24*). Several features make densoviruses potentially effective biological control agents against cockroaches: They tend to be highly host-specific, they infect most tissues of their hosts, they do not appear capable of infecting vertebrates, and they resist extreme environmental conditions. The tendency of cockroaches to aggregate and the ready movement of materials among them should facilitate the use of *Bg*DNV in attractive baits to initiate and maintain epizootics.

Chemical Approaches

Wickham (*25*; see also other reviews in *19*) and Braness (*26*) reviewed the active ingredients and formulations that are used to control household pests, and Ebeling (*27*) compiled a thorough review of inorganic insecticides used against the German cockroach.

Insecticide Sprays

"Space" treatments with various aerosol dispensers usually deploy nonresidual insecticides, such as synergized pyrethrins, allethrin, esfenvalerate, and resemethrin. Nevertheless, residual pyrethroids (e.g., cypermethrin) and insect growth regulators (e.g., hydroprene) are often used in consumer products, such as total-release aerosols ("foggers"). Nonresidual formulations, most containing pyrethrins, are also used by pest control technicians as flushing agents and by consumers in direct application to the pest. The efficacy of such treatments against the German cockroach is poorly documented.

For several decades, both consumers and pest control technicians have favored applications of broad-spectrum insecticides with long residual activity because the insecticides can be applied relatively rapidly and this approach allowed for longer intervals between treatments. Even in the context of better targeted approaches, such as the spot or "crack and crevice" treatments, the usual practice often consists of an initial application at a high rate, followed by regularly scheduled applications at lower rates. Broadcast, or general treatments of surfaces and baseboards with carbamates (bendiocarb, propoxur), organophosphates (acephate, chlorpyrifos, diazinon, propetamphos), abamectin, and pyrethroids were common practices into the early 1990s. Recently, however, such treatments, especially with carbamate and organophosphate insecticides, have declined due to federal regulations (e.g., U.S. Food Quality Protection Act of 1996), insecticide resistance, and the development of highly effective bait formulations (below). Nevertheless, high-volume perimeter applications of pyrethroids, fipronil, chlorfenapyr, and neonicotinoids are used as residual barriers to control or repel various outdoor pests, including cockroaches, even though little data are available in support of the efficacy such treatments.

Crack-and-crevice spray applications utilize the same insecticides and formulations as do broadcast sprays. However, these applications use much less insecticide and they rationally target only cockroach aggregations and potential shelters. Also, crack-and-crevice approaches are not limited to spray formulations, as baits and dusts are also most efficacious when applied to cracks and crevices.

Though highly efficacious against *B. germanica*, residual application of powdered boric acid remains an underutilized approach, probably because it can be messy to dispense and its efficacy is slow compared to most other insecticides. Nevertheless, because boric acid has a very good safety record for mammals, we tested its efficacy against German cockroach infestations in farrowing rooms of a swine farm and compared it to the efficacy of cyfluthrin, a residual pyrethroid insecticide commonly used for cockroach control (*17*). Overall, boric acid dust and cyfluthrin spray treatments had comparable efficacy, but boric acid is less expensive and there are no known cases of pest resistance to it. We further showed, under similar field conditions, that boric acid significantly synergized the pathology of the fungus *Metarhizium anisopliae* against the German cockroach (*28*). Although boric acid dust can be used as an adequate alternative to conventional insecticides to control German cockroach infestations, its adoption into integrated cockroach management programs has been significantly constrained by technical limitations (e.g., expensive dusters) and potential human exposure and respiratory health risks associated with dust inhalation.

Insecticide Baits

The German cockroach must feed before molting to the next stage, and food intake and reproduction are intimately linked in adult females (*29*) suggesting that baits should provide efficacious pest management, especially where food resources are limited. Indeed, a major shift has occurred in cockroach control in the last two decades, from residual sprays to gels and containerized baits (bait stations) (Figure 2). Insecticide baits can be placed in delimited zones and they reduce potential environmental contamination. Some baits may be used almost anywhere including sensitive areas such as food processing and preparation areas, hospitals, and biomedical laboratories. Because cockroaches tend to ingest much larger amounts of insecticide than they would otherwise absorb from a residual spray, and efficacious baits tend to kill more slowly, the insecticide, along with potentially toxic metabolites may be defecated or excreted before the cockroach dies, facilitating horizontal transfer of the active ingredient within cockroach aggregations, and potentially secondary mortality.

Paradoxically, while the number of active ingredients and the diversity of their modes of action has slowed for residual insecticides, which are mainly an outcome of discovery programs that target agricultural pests, the assortment of active ingredients and modes of action in cockroach baits continue to increase. Abamectin, acetamiprid, boric acid, fipronil, hydramethylnon, imidacloprid, indoxacarb, and sulfluramid are some actives used in baits, and others, including other neonicotinoids, ryanodine receptor activators, and spinosyns are some new materials being considered against cockroaches. It will be interesting to determine whether the comparative efficacy of these new chemistries is due to low repellency, efficacy at lower dosages, different modes of action, lack of resistance, delayed activity, or the effects of secondary mortality.

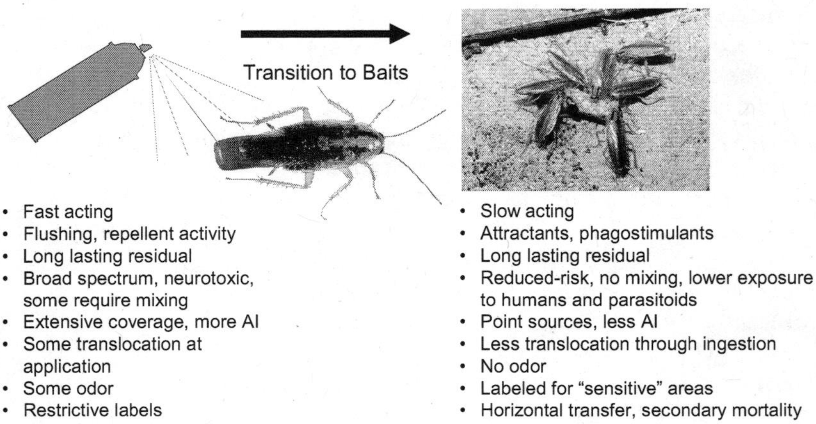

Figure 2. *Comparison of characteristics of spray-based formulations of residual insecticides (left) and reduced-risk bait formulations (right) for German cockroach control. A gravid female is shown (center, with egg case at left) and adults feeding (right).*

Moisture is a limiting resource for cockroaches, and it is likely that gel formulations of baits increase the attraction, acceptability, and efficacy of baits. In addition, unlike containerized bait stations that contain pastes or solid bait matrices, gel baits are dispensed in many more locations that are in close proximity to cockroach aggregations, probably further enhancing their efficacy. Given the superior efficacy of gel baits, it is surprising, however, that liquid baits have not been studied for cockroach control. We evaluated the effectiveness of borate-sugar-water liquid baits in choice and no-choice assays against the German cockroach. Boric acid was more effective than sodium tetraborate or disodium octaborate tetrahydrate, and aqueous solutions containing mixtures of up to 2% boric acid and up to 1 M of several inexpensive sugars (fructose, glucose, maltose, and sucrose) provided rapid and mortality of German cockroaches (*30*). Subsequent trials with liquid baits consisting of 1 or 2% boric acid and 0.5 M sucrose showed that these formulations effectively reduced cockroach infestations in a swine farm nursery (*31*). This approach, however, has not been used in residential settings.

Despite the dramatic rise in bait use, and the indisputably higher efficacy of baits than residual sprays, the basis for selecting an insecticide or a formulation for use in the indoor environment is often less rooted in efficacy and more related to inventories, costs, ease of application, odor, residual material (e.g., tank mix) from a previous application, or consumer preferences.

Horizontal Transfer and Secondary Kill

Certain features of the ecology and reproductive physiology of the German cockroach may constrain the efficacy of bait formulations. For example, females spend most of their adult life in a gravid state during which they feed little and only intermittently (*32*); therefore, baits might be less effective against such females. Likewise, early instar *B. germanica* nymphs forage much less than older nymphs and adults (*33*), and this might reduce the efficacy of insecticidal baits, especially because early instars comprise a large fraction of cockroach populations. Careful placement of baits near cockroach aggregations may alleviate this problem of differential foraging. Another approach is to employ foraging individuals to deliver insecticide or pathogens to non-foraging cockroaches. In principle, this strategy would function best in gregarious or social insects and would require slow-acting insecticides so that foraging insects could return to the aggregation or nest before becoming immobilized by the insecticide.

Silverman et al. (*34*) proposed that German cockroaches redistribute ingested hydramethylnon from baits within aggregations and concluded from translocation assays of radio-labeled hydramethylnon in small cages that coprophagy played a major role in this process. Using assays that differentially excluded nymphs or adults from feeding on insecticide baits, Kopanic and Schal (*35*) quantified the relative contributions of direct (ingestion of bait) and indirect (ingestion of insecticide-laden feces) routes of insecticide uptake in large cages in the laboratory and in field populations. Exclusion of adult females from baits was associated with low mortality of 1st instars, suggesting that under normal conditions high neonate mortality could be attributed primarily to adult-mediated horizontal toxicant transfer through feces. In contrast, mortality of 2nd instars was high and significantly less dependent on adult foraging, suggesting a shift to active foraging (i.e., direct ingestion of bait) during the 2nd stadium. These results are consistent with our understanding of the adaptive benefits of coprophagy in the German cockroach. Starved 1st instars survive significantly longer with access to conspecific feces than when deprived of feces (*36*). In contrast, 2nd instars provided adult feces survived only marginally longer than starved counterparts, showing that coprophagy is stage-specific, as predicted from the bait transfer experiments of Kopanic and Schal (*35*). It appears that the benefit accrues from undigested nutrients in conspecific feces, more than from a symbiotic association with microbes, because nymphs given female feces were more likely to molt into the 2nd stadium than nymphs given male feces, and 1st instars that were fed the feces of adults that had been maintained on a high protein diet survived longer than other cohorts fed the feces of adults that had been maintained on medium (22.5%) and low (5%) protein diets (*36*).

Other bait active ingredients are also horizontally transferred among cockroaches, but the mechanisms may differ, depending on their modes of action and speed of kill. When adult cockroaches were fed boric acid, chlorpyrifos, fipronil, or hydramethylnon in either small or large cages, exposure to the corpses and feces killed all 1st instars and most 2nd instars (*37*). However, when the dead cockroaches were removed from the large arenas and replaced with new cockroaches (i.e., in the absence of cannibalism and necrophagy), only residues of slow-acting hydramethylnon killed most of the nymphs and adults, whereas residues of fast acting insecticides (chlorpyrifos and fipronil) killed fewer nymphs and adults, even when the concentrations of chlorpyrifos and hydramethylnon were equivalent; abamectin baits failed to cause significant mortality in cockroaches that contacted the residues. It is possible that the relatively high concentration of hydramethylnon in the bait (2.15%) and its apparent stability in the digestive tract and feces contribute to the efficacy of hydramethylnon in secondary kill.

Buczkowski and Schal (*38*) evaluated the effects of three different methods of delivering fipronil to adult male German cockroaches on secondary mortality in nymphs and adults. Topical application with an LD_{99} dose (5 ng) was the least effective method for subsequent secondary kill, followed by exposure to residual fipronil deposits on a glass surface, which resulted in some mortality of early instars. Ingested fipronil bait was most effectively translocated, however, and caused high mortality of untreated adults and nymphs, even when compared to an equivalent amount of topically applied fipronil (25 ng). Because fipronil has high contact activity, the mechanisms that cause secondary kill may include contact with fipronil-contaminated substrates as well as ingestion of excreted residues and cannibalism of bait-fed cockroaches. However, unlike hydramethylnon, which is translocated primarily through coprophagy, fipronil is excreted mainly during onset of the paralytic symptoms, and most of the radio-labeled fipronil is excreted orally (*39*). Time-lapse video analysis further showed that 1st instars were attracted to these excretions, imbibed the liquid exudates, and died – a process termed emetophagy, which may constitute an important mechanism by which fast-acting, emetogenic insecticides are disseminated within cockroach populations (*39*). Buczkowski et al. (*40*) further extended these ideas to indoxacarb and tertiary kill, showing that ingested indoxacarb was most effectively translocated when the recipients interacted with freshly symptomatic donors in the absence of alternative food.

The extensive findings from laboratory assays would suggest that horizontal transfer of bait active ingredients might contribute significantly to bait efficacy in the field. Although Kopanic and Schal (*35*) concluded, based on limited field results, that "horizontal toxicant transfer is a key factor in suppression of cockroach pest populations," and horizontal transfer of bait is a heavily marketed phenomenon (e.g., as secondary and tertiary kill, domino effect, exponential control), no follow-up studies have been conducted in the field to critically evaluate the magnitude and significance of bait transfer in cockroach control.

Integrated Cockroach Management

The indoor environment is highly conducive to implementation of a variety of approaches and tools, including use of photolabile active ingredients and physical and structural modifications to manipulate pest behavior and their spatial distribution. However, despite of the plethora of available options, cockroach suppression still relies heavily upon multiple applications of broad-spectrum insecticides to individual units (apartments, rooms in a nursing home, etc.), with little appreciation of the movement patterns of cockroaches. Often, integration of management options consists of mixing several related insecticides. But recent regulatory emphasis on IPM in school systems has resulted in greater emphasis on education and communication among researchers, extension personnel, consultants, pest control technicians, and the concerned public. Concomitantly, several recent studies have documented the superiority of integrated pest management approaches over calendar-based conventional spraying in both schools and residences.

Miller and Meek (*41*) compared the long-term costs and efficacy of a monthly baseboard and crack-and-crevice treatment with spray and dust formulations to a monitoring-based IPM treatment that involved vacuuming of apartments followed by monthly or quarterly applications of baits and insect growth regulator in Virginia public housing residences. The expenses associated with the IPM treatment—the costs of technician time and product applied—were higher than for the conventional treatment, but it was also much more effective. Indeed, trap catch data suggested that the conventional treatment had little effect on the cockroach populations over the course of a year.

A similar study, also comparing IPM and conventional approaches, but in North Carolina elementary schools, reached different conclusions. Although the IPM services were significantly more time-consuming, and therefore incurred higher costs associated with labor, the overall costs of the two types of treatments were similar, as was their efficacy of cockroach control (*42*). However, environmental residues of acephate, chlorpyrifos, and propetamphos were higher in swab samples taken in the conventionally treated schools.

Allergen Mitigation Strategies

Seven *B. germanica*-produced allergens have been identified and characterized, and aqueous extracts of several cockroach tissues, including the intestinal tract Malpighian tubules, ovaries, ootheca, exuvia, and feces, are allergenic to sensitized individuals. Gore and Schal (*43*) provide an extensive review of the molecular biology, tissue distribution, and allergenicity of each allergen, as well as sampling methodology, demographics of cockroach allergen exposure and sensitization, and intervention studies aimed at allergen mitigation in infested homes.

Reduced-Risk Baits: Pivotal Components of Allergen Mitigation

The central tenet of allergic disease and asthma intervention is to minimize exposure through environmental allergen reduction, involving (*a*) suppression of cockroach populations, and (*b*) removal of residual cockroach allergens. Indeed, there is a strong correlation between cockroach allergen concentrations in kitchen dust and German cockroach populations based on trap catches, with $r = 0.73$ for Bla g 1 (*Blattella germanica* allergen 1) and $r = 0.84$ for Bla g 2 (*44*). However, most environmental interventions that used a two-pronged approach of pest control and cleaning failed to attain clinically significant reductions of cockroach allergens in infested homes (see supplemental Table in *43*). Several reasons likely account for these results, including inadequate or lack of monitoring of the cockroach population, infrequent and outdated pest control treatments that resulted in inferior efficacy, and poor resident buy-in and cooperation with the programs.

More recent studies have followed the recognition that extensive cleaning and resident education could not be fully efficacious without highly effective pest control and impartial assessments of the pest population (hence, efficacy of the intervention). A 6-month intervention study in North Carolina combined extensive monitoring-guided and lay-out maps-guided treatments with reduced-risk hydramethylnon gel bait, resident education, and professional cleaning that was also guided by trap catch (*45*). For the first time in an allergen mitigation study, large reductions in the cockroach populations were observed in treatment homes: by month 6, the median trap catch was 0 in each monitored room (kitchen, living room, bed room; 113, 76 and 78, respectively at baseline), trap counts were 0 in 9 kitchens, 11 living rooms, and 12 bedrooms of the 16 homes, and 37.5% of the homes had no trapped cockroaches in any room. The high efficacy of cockroach control was accompanied by significant reductions in cockroach allergen levels below the human sensitization threshold: Bla g 1, a major aeroallergen with up to 77% IgE prevalence among cockroach-allergic individuals (*46*), decreased in concentration (Units per grm dust) from 633 to 24 on kitchen floors (96% reduction), from 25 to 4.3 on living room floors/sofas (83%), from 46 to 7.3 on bedroom floors (84%), and from 6.1 to 1.0 in bedroom beds (84% reduction) (*45*).

The success of this intervention led us to examine which of the three intervention tactics was key to the observed effects, because the two physical interventions were not equally deployable: whole home cleaning was substantially more expensive and intrusive than pest control. Therefore, a 6-month continuation of the Arbes et al. (*45*) study, crossed-over the non-intervention control homes to an intensive, targeted insecticide bait treatment, while the intervention homes continued to receive this treatment on an intermittent, as-needed basis; neither treatment group received cleaning or resident education and untreated control homes were not included (*47*). The results showed that pest control alone resulted in large reductions in the cockroach populations, but surprisingly, it also brought about highly significant reductions in Bla g 1 levels. The mean Bla g 1 concentrations decreased from 287 to 14.4 on kitchen floors (95% reduction), from 28.8 to 5.6 on living room floors/sofas (81%), from 26.7 to 4.7 on bedroom floors (82%), and from 7.2 to

2.4 for beds (67% reduction); similar results were seen for the allergen Bla g 2 (*47*).

Baits have become a pivotal tool in cockroach control. Wang and Bennett (*48*) compared a bait-alone intervention with an IPM approach (cockroaches flushed and vacuumed, sticky traps deployed, educational materials delivered, and fipronil- and hydramethylnon-containing baits) on a building-wide basis in public housing in Indiana. No allergen measurements were conducted. Of 5 post-treatment evaluations during a 7 month period, cockroach control was significantly more efficacious in IPM apartments in only 2 evaluations (1 and 4 months after initial treatment), but the 1-month evaluation appeared to be aberrant due to a decline in efficacy from 48% at week 2 to 18% at week 4 and then up to 96% at week 8, and the efficacy at month 4 was 100% (IPM) and 96.4% (bait only). Although Wang and Bennett (*48*) conclude that "IPM is a more sustainable method of population reduction" the cost of IPM was significantly higher than that of the bait treatment and the benefits appeared to be nominal.

The impressive efficacy of baits alone (*47*, *48*), coupled with the fact that baits constitute a major component of any IPM program of cockroach control, highlight an important public policy implication—under the constraints of tight public housing budgets, most of the intervention effort should be invested in bait-based eradication of cockroach infestations. Extensive cleaning is clearly required to remove residual allergens, but this rather costly effort is best reserved as a follow-up to cockroach eradication.

In a commentary about the Arbes et al. (*45*) article, Eggleston (*49*) stated: "[it] is a model of the sort of difficult, well-planned, and well-executed clinical research that will move the field of environmental avoidance forward. It represents what is technically called an efficacy trial in that the investigators chose to apply the treatment with as little reliance on the adherence of the families participating as possible. This is as opposed to an effectiveness trial that would apply the treatment as it might be applied in clinical practice or by a public health department, usually relying on participant adherence." In light of the general disappointing results of most interventions involving professional pest control (see *43* for a summary), Eggelston's appeal for an effectiveness trail was well founded.

To evaluate the effectiveness of professional pest control in cockroach allergen mitigation, we used untreated control homes and two intervention groups of homes in North Carolina: one treated with insecticide baits applied by research personnel following previously established protocols (lay-out maps, sticky traps, whole-home baiting), and the other provided with professional pest control (*50*). Once again, the intensive, targeted approach was highly efficacious, reducing the median cockroach trap catch from 426.5 to 0 within 6 months, and cockroaches apparently were eliminated in 62.5% of the homes. From baseline to month 12, mean Bla g 1 concentrations decreased from 64.2 to 5.6 in kitchens (91.3% reduction), 10.6 to 1.1 in living rooms (89.6%), 10.7 to 1.9 on bedroom floors (82.2%), but only 3.6 to 2.3 in the bed (36.1% reduction). In contrast, homes treated by commercial technicians showed a much smaller decline in the cockroach population from 308.5 at baseline to 56.0 at month 6 (81.6% reduction, 1 of 17 homes with 0 trap catch) and Bla g 1 levels decreased from

66.9 to 43.0 in the kitchen (35.7% reduction), 14.3 to 5.7 in the living room (60.1%), 17.3 to 7.2 on the bedroom floor (58.4%), and from 5.5 to 1.9 in the bed (65.4% reduction). However, these changes were not significant compared with the untreated control homes (*50*). Although the contract-based commercial pest control was substantially less effective at reducing cockroach infestations and allergens, it was comparable to previously reported environmental interventions that employed pest control technicians (see *43* for review).

These results suggest that the relationship between the cockroach population and allergen concentration in a home is not linear—particularly during the decline in the cockroach population that occurs during pest control operations. The actual relationship may be exponential, such that a very large reduction in the cockroach infestation is needed to achieve significant reductions in the allergen level. The real shape of this relationship will have to await experimental evidence with a much higher sample size. But, if correct, the implication of this model is that some pest control practices may be acceptable to the consumer because they reduce the cockroach population, but because allergen levels remain above threshold values these practices may be clinically inferior.

Whole-Home vs. Partial Intervention

Sever et al. (*50*) consider some of the technical, operational, and economic factors that may underlie the differences between efficacy and effectiveness trials. We speculated that the spatial distribution of the pest control efforts within homes might be important. Most commercial and consumer-based pest control, as well as academic field efficacy trials, treat only the kitchens, pantries and bathrooms, whereas we (*45*, *47*, *50*) treated whole homes. The rationale for our approach was that cockroaches in low-income NC homes are distributed throughout the home, including living rooms and bedrooms (Figure 3). Moreover, analysis of allergens in homes has shown that while cockroach allergen concentration is highest on the kitchen floor, the concentration on the living room floor is 67.4% as high, and allergen concentration on the bedroom floor is 55.9% that of kitchen dust (*51*), and asthmatic children are more likely to be more intimate contact longer with bedroom dust than kitchen dust. It is important to note that these values do not address allergen load in various rooms, that is, the total amount of allergen contained in all dust in the room.

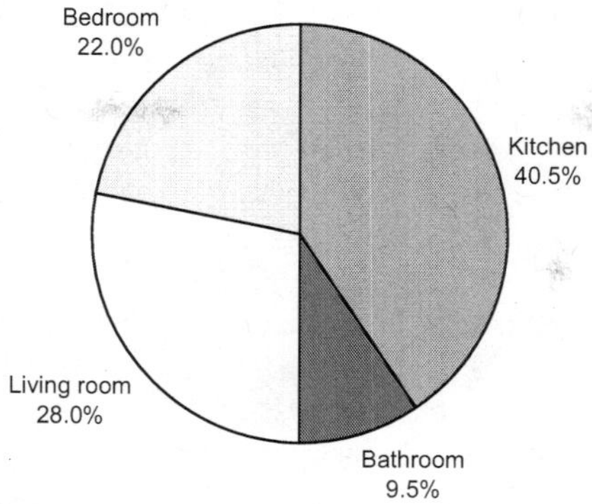

Figure 3. *Distribution of cockroaches among four rooms of 41 apartments in North Carolina. Four traps were deployed in each room, except the bathroom, which received only two traps. For this analysis, we consider percentage trapped cockroaches per trap per room.*

A comparison, in progress, of baiting whole homes with indoxacarb bait versus baiting the kitchen and bathroom only with the same amount of bait suggests that when total trap catch is considered (*a*) a significantly faster decline in cockroaches is evident in whole home treatments within 7 days after the initial treatment, and (*b*) differences between the two interventions persist for at least 3 months, to the end of the trial (Santangelo et al., unpublished). As expected, we found no differences in the magnitude of the reductions in cockroach trap catches over time in the two interventions, but much faster and larger reductions were evident in the living rooms and bedrooms of the whole home treatments. Allergen samples from this work are being analyzed.

Interestingly, Wang and Bennett (*48*) were able to bait apartments over a 29 week period in a cumulative median time of 22 min per apartment, whereas our baiting efforts required at least 45 min per apartment for the initial treatment alone. While these differences might be attributable to different levels of sanitation, clutter, apartment sizes, resident cooperation, and cockroach population sizes, we suspect, again, that they relate to different spatial distributions of the baiting programs. Wang and Bennett (48) treated kitchens, pantries and bathrooms only, whereas we (*45*, *47*, *50*) treated the whole home. Using 10 microsatellite loci, we recently genotyped German cockroaches from 18 populations in Raleigh. Our preliminary results indicate that cockroaches collected in various rooms within a single apartment are panmictic, i.e., represent a single population, whereas cockroaches collected from different residences– even adjacent apartments – were genetically differentiated (Crissman et al., unpublished). Because dispersal and gene flow occur more often within apartments than between them, and various rooms in the home can be infested with cockroaches (Figure 3), it seems sensible to treat the whole residence as a target of cockroach control efforts.

Outcomes of Interventions

A major uncertainty in allergen mitigation studies is the fate of the allergens. Extensive professional cleaning, even with denaturing agents, has generally resulted in only mediocre allergen reductions whwn pest control is substandard or unreported (see review: *43*). In contrast, highly efficacious cockroach control, with or without cleaning, dramatically reduced allergen levels. Obviously, only allergen on accessible (sampled) surfaces was reduced (i.e., vacuumed and sieved for ELISA, see *52*) – the allergen load in inaccessible voids and behind and under appliances and kitchen cabinets has not changed. We suggest that as few or no cockroaches remain to forage and defecate, less allergen is detected on exposed surfaces. A major uncertainty is whether the sampled surfaces best represent clinically relevant allergen concentrations, or if the large allergen reservoirs that remain inaccessible (see Figure 1) contribute to the aeroallergen population. Gore and Schal (*43*) review allergen sampling methodology and the potential health outcomes of successful interventions.

The global success of *B. germanica* has been associated with more constant environmental control and poor maintenance of structures, inferior sanitation, relatively inefficacious and difficult to apply spray insecticides, and a vast array of consumer products of questionable efficacy – especially when improperly deployed. An irony of insecticide discovery is that as biologically and genomically-inspired design, artificial networks, combinatorial chemistry, and high-throughput *in vitro* screening have become more available, market and regulatory forces have acted to slow the pace of introduction of new insecticides with new modes of action against agricultural pests. Hopefully, the recent economic and regulatory successes of bait formulations, as well as their superior efficacy, will continue to fuel a trend counter to that of insecticide discovery in agriculture.

Acknowledgements

I thank several recent collaborators, particularly Darryl Zeldin, Samuel Arbes and Michelle Sever (NIEHS), and Herman Mitchell (Rho). Richard Santangello provided excellent technical support, and recent graduate students and post-doctoral fellows contributed to the ideas and projects described herein. Recent research in this area was supported in part by USDA-NRI (2004-35302-14880), USDA-RAMP (2005-51101-02388), and the Blanton J. Whitmire endowment at North Carolina State University.

References

1. Platts-Mills, T. A. E.; Wheatley, L. M.; Aalberse, R. C. *Curr. Opin. Immunol.* **1998**, *10*, 634–639.
2. Dey, A. N.; Bloom, B. *Vital Health Stat. 10* **2005**, *223*, 1–87.
3. Weiss, K. B.; Sullivan, S. D. *J. Allergy Clin. Immunol.* **2001**, *107*, 3–8.
4. Arbes, S. J. Jr.; Gergen, P. J.; Elliott, L.; Zeldin, D. C. *J. Allergy Clin. Immunol.* **2005**, *116*, 377–383.
5. Rosenstreich, D. L.; Eggleston, P.; Kattan, M.; Baker, D.; Slavin, R. G. et al. *N. Engl. J. Med.* **1997**, *336*, 1356–1363.
6. Gelber, L. E.; Seltzer, L. H.; Bouzoukis, J. K.; Pollart, S. M.; Chapman, M. D.; Platts-Mills, T. A. E. *Am. Rev. Respir. Dis.* **1993**, *147*, 573–578.
7. Gold, D. R.; Burge, H. A.; Carey, V.; Milton, D. K.; Platts-Mills, T.; Weiss, S. T. *Am. J. Respir. Crit. Care Med.* **1999**, *160*, 227–236.
8. Brenner, R. J. In *Understanding and Controlling the German Cockroach*; Rust, M. K.; Owens, J. M.; Reierson, D. A., Eds. 1995. Oxford Univ. Press: NY, 1995, pp 77–92.
9. Cloarec, A.; Rivault, C.; Fontaine, F.; Le Guyader, A. *Epidemiol. Infect.* **1992**, *109*, 483–490.
10. Rivault, C;. Cloarec, A.; Le Guyader, A. *Epidemiol. Infect.* **1993**, *110*, 317–325.
11. Moon, H. W.; Hoffman, L. J.; Cornick, N. A.; Booher, S. L.; Bosworth, B. T. *J. Vet. Diagn. Invest.* **1999**, *11*, 557–560.
12. Zurek, L.; Schal, C. *Vet. Microbiol.* **2004**, *101*, 263–267.
13. Whyatt, R. M.; Barr, D. B.; Camann, D. E.; Kinney, P. L.; Barr, J. R.; Andrews, H. F. et al. *Environ. Health Perspect.* **2003**, *111*, 749–756.
14. Berkowitz, G. S.; Wetmur, J. G.; Birman-Deych, E.; Obel, J.; Lapinski, R. H.; Godbold, J. H. et al. *Environ. Health Perspect.* **2004**, *112*, 388–391.
15. Bradman, A.; Whyatt, R. M. *Environ. Health Perspect.* **2005**, *113*, 1092–1099.
16. Rudant, J.; Menegaux, F.; Leverger, G.; Baruchel, A.; Nelken, B.; Bertrand, Y. et al. *Environ. Health Perspect.* **2007**, *115*, 1787–1793.
17. Zurek, L.; Gore, J. C.; Stringham, M. S.; Watson, D. W.; Waldvogel, M. G.; Schal, C. *J. Econ. Entomol.* **2003**, *96*, 1362–1366.
18. Schal, C.; Hamilton, R. *Annu. Rev. Entomol.* **1990**, *35*, 521–551.
19. *Understanding and Controlling the German Cockroach*; Rust, M. K.; Owens, J. M.; Reierson, D. A., Eds. Oxford Univ. Press: NY, 1995, 430 pp.
20. Benson, E. P.; Zungoli, P. A. In *Handbook of Pest Control*; Moreland, D. Ed., Mallis Handbook and Technical Training Co.: Cleveland, OH, 8th ed., pp 122–202.
21. Gold, R. E. In *Understanding and Controlling the German Cockroach*; Rust, M. K.; Owens, J. M.; Reierson, D. A., Eds. Oxford Univ. Press: NY, 1995, pp 325–344.
22. Suiter, D. R. *J. Agric. Entomol.* **1997**, *14*, 259–270.
23. Milner, R. J.; Pereira, R. M. In *Field Manual of Techniques in Invertebrate Pathology*; Lacey, L. A.; Kaya, H. K. Eds. Springer, 2007, pp 695–711.
24. Mukha, D. V.; Chumachenko, A. G.; Dykstra, M. J.; Kurtti, J.; Schal, C. *J. Gen. Virol.* **2006**, *87*, 1567–1575.

25. Wickham, J. C. In *Understanding and Controlling the German Cockroach*; Rust, M. K.; Owens, J. M.; Reierson, D. A., Eds. Oxford Univ. Press: NY, 1995, pp 109–148.
26. Braness, G. In *Handbook of Pest Control*; Moreland, D. Ed., Frazak &Foster Co.: Cleaveland, OH, 8th ed., pp 1061–1101.
27. Ebeling, W. In *Understanding and Controlling the German Cockroach*; Rust, M. K.; Owens, J. M.; Reierson, D. A., Eds. Oxford Univ. Press: NY, 1995, pp 193–230.
28. Zurek, L.; Watson, D. W.; Schal, C. *Biol. Control* **2002**, *23*, 296–302.
29. Schal, C.; Holbrook, G. L.; Bachmann, J. A. S.; Sevala, V. L. *Arch. Insect Biochem. Physiol.* **1997**, *35*, 405–426.
30. Gore, J. C.; Schal, C. *J. Econ. Entomol.* **2004**, *97*, 581–587.
31. Gore J. C.; Zurek, L.; Santangelo, R. G.; Stringham, S. M.; Watson, D. W.; Schal, C. *J. Econ. Entomol.* **2004**, *97*, 715–720.
32. Hamilton, R.; Schal, C. *Ann. Entomol. Soc. Am.* **1988**, *81*, 969–976.
33. Kopanic, R. J., Jr.; Schal, C. *Environ. Entomol.* **1999**, *28*, 431–438.
34. Silverman, J.; Vitale, G. I.; Shapas, T. J. *J. Econ. Entomol.* **1991**, 84, 176–180
35. Kopanic, R. J., Jr.; Schal, C. *J. Econ. Entomo.* **1997**, *90*, 1073–1079.
36. Kopanic, R. J., Jr.; Holbrook, G. L.; Sevala, V.; Schal, C. *Ecol. Entomol.* **2001**, *26*, 154–162.
37. Buczkowski, G.; Kopanic, R. J.; Schal, C. *J. Econ. Entomol.* **2001**, *94*, 1229–1236.
38. Buczkowski, G.; Schal, C. *J. Econ. Entomol.* **2001**, *94*, 680–685.
39. Buczkowski, G.; Schal, C. *Pestic. Biochem. Physiol.* **2001**, *71*, 147–155.
40. Buczkowski, G.; Scherer, C. W.; Bennett, G. W. *J. Econ. Entomol.* **2008**, *101*, 894–901 .
41. Miller, D. M.; Meek, F. *J. Econ. Entomol.* **2004**, *97*, 559–569
42. Williams, G. M.; Linker, H. M.; Waldvogel, M. G.; Leidy, R. B.; Schal, C. *J. Econ. Entomol.* **2005**, *98*, 1275–1283.
43. Gore, J. C.; Schal, C. *Annu. Rev. Entomol.* **2007**, *52*, 439–463.
44. Wang, C.; Abou El-Nour, M. M.; Bennett, G. W. *J. Community Health* **2008**, *33*, 31–39
45. Arbes, S. J., Jr.; Sever, M.; Archer, J.; Long, E. H.; Gore, J. C.; Schal, C.; et al. *J. Allergy Clin. Immunol.* **2003**, *112*, 339–345.
46. Helm, R.; Cockrell, G.; Stanley, J. S.; Brenner, R. J., Burks, W.; Bannon, G. A. *J. Allergy Clin. Immunol.* **1996**, *98*, 172–180
47. Arbes, S. J., Jr.; Sever, M.; Mehta, J.; Gore, J. C.; Schal, C.; Vaughn, B.; et al.. *J. Allergy Clin. Immunol.* **2004**, *113*, 109–114.
48. Wang, C.; Bennett, G. W. *J. Econ. Entomol.* **2006**, *99*, 879–885
49. Eggleston, P. A. *J. Allergy Clin. Immunol.* **2003**, *112*, 265–267.
50. Sever, M. L.; Arbes, S. J., Jr.; Gore, J. C., Jr.; Santangelo, R. G.; Vaughn, B.; Mitchell, H.; et al. *J. Allergy Clin. Immunol.* **2007**, *120*, 849–855.
51. Cohn, R. D.; Arbes, S .J., Jr.; Jaramillo, R.; Reid, L. H.; Zeldin, D. C. Environ. Health Perspect. **2006**, *114*, 522–526
52. Mansour, M.; Lanphear, B.; Hornung, R.; Khoury, J.; Bernstein, D. et al. *Environ. Res.* **2001**, *87*, 37–46

Chapter 8

Current Status of House Dust Mites in Japan and Prospects for Control Agents

Tomoyuki HASHIMOTO

Department of Environmental Biology, Japan Environmental Sanitation Center, Kawasaki, Japan

Mite infestations in school and home environments in Japan were investigated during 2005–2006. The mite numbers in summer exceeded the thresholds set by Japanese ministries (Ministry of Education, Sports, Culture, Science and Technology and the Ministry of Health and Welfare). *Dermatophagoides* spp. were dominant in schools and residences with more than 80% average presence. The acaricidal efficacy of several compounds was evaluated. Phenyl salicylate and benzyl benzoate indicated acaricidal efficacy by continuous contact. Etoxazole suppressed hatchability of the *D. farinae* eggs and exerted growth-regulatory effects. Amidoflumet was most effective against *D. farinae*. Amidoflumet treatment combined with vacuuming once a week caused a drastic reduction of live mites within 8 days. However, the reduction of mite allergen was not obvious. Thus, more frequent vacuuming might be required to reduce the allergen load.

House dust mites (HDMs), including *Dermatophagoides farinae* and *D. pteronyssinus* are detected in all human habitations. These ubiquitous mites can sensitize humans and cause asthma, rhinitis, and atopic dermatitis by means of allergens derived from their feces (Der 1) or bodies (Der 2). The HDM allergen is medically important in Japan, especially in the case of children (1, 2).

Information about mite infestation is indispensable for protection from exposure to the allergen. Therefore, many studies on mite fauna, mite population, and mite allergen levels in houses (3, 4), schools (5), transportation (6), and public facilities (7, 8) have been carried out in Japan. In order to reduce the probability of exposure to the HDM, allergen avoidance and removal of the allergen are recommended (9). As a part of the allergen control strategy, a number of anti-mite techniques have been developed. Currently, several efficient acaricides have become available in Japan, and the use of control agents has also been considered as an anti-mite intervention.

This paper describes the current status of HDM infestations in school and home environments in Japan and reports the acaricidal efficacy of several compounds.

Mite infestation in school and home environments in Japan

Mite infestation in human dwellings is a public health concern in Japan. The mite density fluctuates depending on indoor environments such as the structure of the house (10), the indoor climate (11, 12), and human activity (13).

Changes in the flooring materials particularly influenced mite distribution. Most tatami mats currently consist of an artificial core such as Styrofoam, sandwiched between a thick paperboard, instead of a natural straw core. Consequently, outbreaks caused by *Tyrophagus putrescentiae*, Glycyphagidae spp., and Cheyletidae spp. seem to be decreased (14). Furthermore, wood has become a more popular choice of flooring material in newly built residences in Japan than tatami or carpets. Replacing the carpeted floor with the wooden floor during renovations not only affected dust accumulation but also mite distribution (15). Thus, mite infestation is generally dependent on the flooring materials.

In order to improve the quality of life, the Ministry of Health and Welfare (MHW) published guidelines for the control of HDMs in 1999 (16). These guidelines proposed threshold values of mite infestation for different flooring and bedding materials in residences. These values are as follows: 100 mites/m^2 for tatami, 300 mites or 1μg of Der 1/m^2 for carpeted floors, 100 mites or 1μg Der 1/m^2 for bedding, and 10 mites or 0.005 μg of Der 1/m^2 for wooden floors.

The percentage of asthmatic children has been increasing in all types of schools (Figure 1). Particularly in elementary schools, an increase of

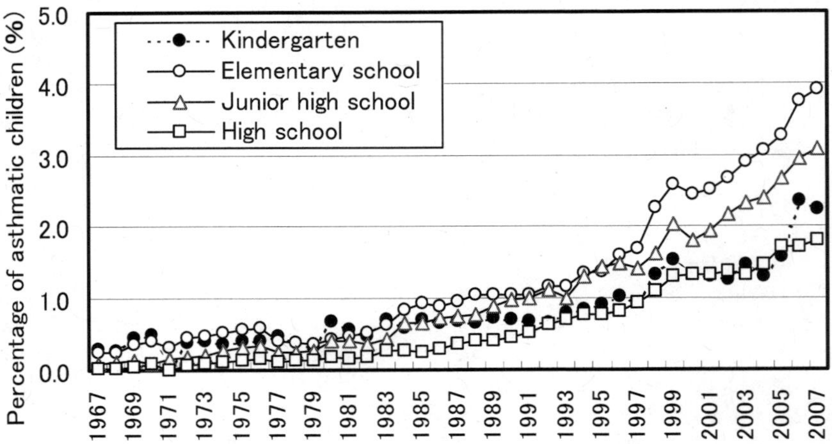

Figure 1 Fluctuation in the percentage of asthmatic school children in Japan. (Data obtained from reference 17).

approximately 4 % was observed in 2007 (17). In view of these tendencies, the Ministry of Education, Culture, Sports, Science and Technology (MEXT) has mandated an annual inspection of HDMs in classroom carpet and infirmary beddings since 2004, and the threshold for mite infestation, beyond which interventions against HDMs becomes necessary, was fixed at 100 mites/m^2 (18).

As worldwide standards, the risk factors suggested by the World Health Organization (WHO) (19) have often been quoted in previous studies. In the WHO proposal, a level of 2 μg Der 1/g dust (equivalent to 100 mites) is regarded as a risk factor for sensitization and the development of asthma. A higher level of 10 μg Der 1/g dust (or 500 mites/g of dust) is considered a major risk factor for the development of acute asthma in mite-sensitized individuals. However, the WHO index is different from that of the Japanese ministries. Most previous investigations conducted in Japan have expressed the mite population in terms of number of mites per gram of dust. Unfortunately however, many studies have not provided information about the weight of the dust and the sample size. Therefore, it has been difficult to compare the mite populations reported in previous studies with the thresholds set by the Japanese ministries.

The author has examined samples obtained from Japanese schools in Tokyo and Kanagawa during 2005–2006.

Mite infestations in school environments

In an inspection conducted in July 2005 in Tokyo, house dust was collected from the floors and beddings in classrooms, libraries, infirmaries, computer rooms, etc., of 29 schools by an electric vacuum cleaner (20). The mites were isolated from the dust by using the saturated saline floating method (3). The inspection revealed that in only 6 of the 146 samples (4.1%) the number of mites exceeded the threshold (100 mites/m^2) set by the MEXT. On the other hand, in 56 samples (38.4%), the number of mites exceeded the value of 100 mites/g dust, which is a risk factor for sensitization to asthma (19), while in 14 samples (9.6%), the number of mites exceeded the value of 500 mites/g of dust, which is a major risk factor for acute asthma. *D. farinae* was the dominant species, occurring at rates greater than 80% in all materials, excepting tatami. Thus, achieving the WHO threshold was supposedly more difficult than achieving the MEXT threshold. The mean numbers of mites per square meter and per gram of dust are compared in Table 1.

Table 1 Comparison of numbers of mites in each material

Material	*No. of Samples*	*Mean weight of collected dust (mg/m^2)*	*Mean no. of mites (/m^2)*	*Mean no. of mites (/g dust)*
Carpets	47	239	24	117
Wooden floor	34	181	9	120
Tatami	11	186	41	374
Bedding	54	63	14	233

(Data obtained from reference 20)

In another inspection conducted in the Kanagawa Prefecture, in March and August 2006, mites on the surface of carpeted floors and infirmary beddings in 10 schools were detected by using the adhesive lint roller method (21). Although the number of mites in the 30 samples collected in March did not exceed the MEXT threshold, this number in 15 of the 35 samples collected in August (42.9%) exceeded the threshold. The mean (± SD) mite numbers in the bedding and carpet were 97 ± 88 and 173 ± 219 mites/m^2, respectively. House dust was also collected by using a vacuum cleaner. The HDM allergen was extracted in phosphate-buffered saline (PBS) and measured using the enzyme-linked immunosorbent assay (ELISA). In August, the mean amounts of the Der 1 allergen increased to more than 3.0 μg/m^2 in both the beddings and carpets (Figure 2). In this investigation too, *Dermatophagoides* mites predominated over the mite fauna of most schools (Table 2) (22).

Since there are only a few carpeted classrooms in Japanese schools, it is considered that the probability of exposure to the mite allergen in schools is

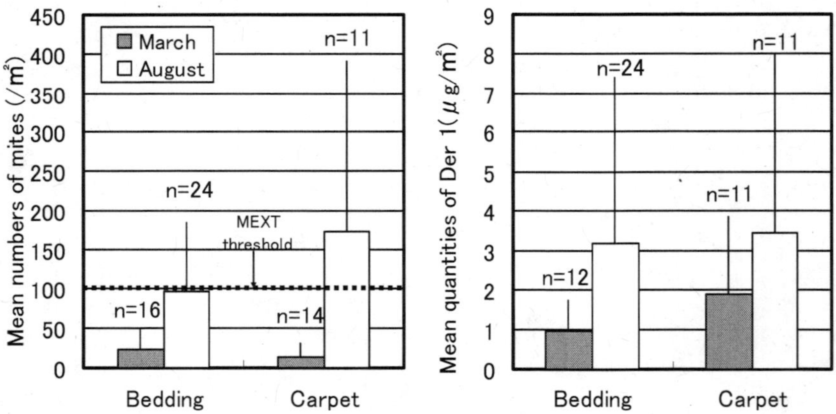

Figure 2 The number of mites and quantity of Der 1 allergen in schools in the Kanagawa Prefecture. (Data obtained from reference 22). The threshold for the number of mites was determined by the MEXT in 2004.

Table 2 Dominance of *Dermatophagoides spp.* in the mite fauna of school environments.

	No.of samples	*Percentage of Dermatophagoides spp.* among total number of mites*
Bedding – March	16	90.2%
Bedding – August	24	92.6%
Carpet – March	14	95.6%
Carpet – August	11	97.3%

**D. farinae* and *D. pteronyssinus* were included.

(Data obtained from reference 22)

lesser than that at home. However, it is expected that the percentage of asthmatic school children will increase, and that allergy to HDM will also be an important problem in the future. In order to reduce the exposure risk, the HDMs and their allergens should be removed to the maximum extent possible.

Mite infestations in home environments

In 2006, mite infestation in dwellings was also investigated (23). This investigation targeted only houses with wooden floors in the living rooms or bedrooms and included more than 200 residences from all over Japan. The mites were captured by the adhesive lint roller method in winter and summer. Moreover, house dust in from 19 residences of the targeted residences was collected in all 4 seasons by using a vacuum cleaner, and the quantity of HDM allergen was determined using ELISA. The results showed that the mean mite number in summer was 7-fold greater than that in winter, and that the numbers of mites in 49% of the investigated houses in summer exceeded the MHW threshold (Table 3). The proportion of *Dermatophagoides* mites to total number of mites fluctuated between 71–86% among seasons.

Table 3 Mite infestation of wooden floors in residences.

Season	*No.of houses*	*Mean no. of mites (/m²)*	*Mean no. of Dermatophagoides mites (/m²)* [% of total]	*No.of houses with >10 mites/m²** [% of total]
Winter	274	3.8 ± 10.9	2.7 ± 7.6 [71]	27 [10]
Summer	221	28.0 ± 55.9	24.1 ± 50.6 [86]	109 [49]

*: Threshold for the wooden floor proposed by the MHW in 1999.

Regarding the HDM allergen, the mean allergen quantity gradually increased from winter to autumn. The mean Der 1 quantities in the selected residences were higher than 0.005 $\mu g/m^2$ in all seasons (Figure 3). It was considered that one of the factors responsible for this result was the weight of the dust, because the mean weight of the dust collected in each season also increased from winter to autumn. A significantly ($p < 0.01$; n = 89) high correlation was observed between the quantities of both the allergens (Der 1 and Der 2) and the weight of the dust (Figure 4). This investigation revealed that although the wooden floor occasionally harbored many mites, the infestation of beddings might be considerably more severe as they are the most important breeding source for HDMs.

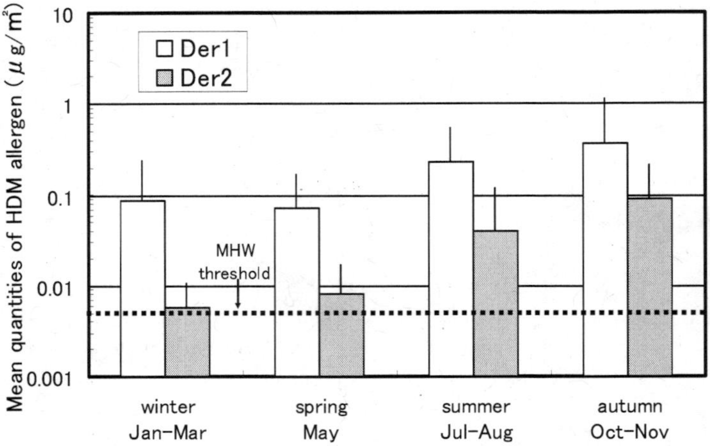

Figure 3 Mean quantities of mite allergen in the residences examined. The threshold value for the wooden floors was proposed by the MHW in 1999.

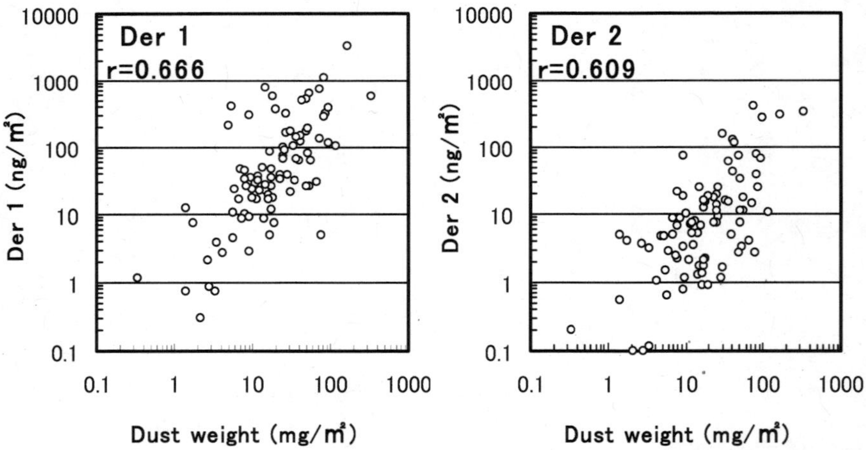

Figure 4 Correlation between dust weight and the quantity of the HDM allergen. r: Spearman's rank correlation coefficient. (n = 89)

Control agents for house dust mites

In order to prevent exposure to mite allergens, many measures have been taken. For instance, introduction of wooden flooring (24) and impermeable bed covers (25) prevent the mite infestation. In addition, large-sized washing machines and high-powered vacuum cleaners are useful devices, which can be used to eliminate HDMs and reduce the accumulation of HDM allergens (26). We can physically eliminate mites from bedding or flooring by using these devices after infestation.

Despite the advances in chemical-free strategies, the chemical treatment has not become the principal choice for the elimination of the HDM allergens. One of the reasons for this situation is that the control agents may kill HDMs, but their allergens can be eliminated by acaricide treatment alone. After acaricide treatment, the removal of the carcasses and feces is eventually required. Second, the active ingredient of the control agents does not penetrate to the microhabitats of the HDMs. Carpet piles, bed covers, and tatami surfaces occasionally become barriers that prevent the contact between the chemical agent and the HDMs. Besides, not only allergic patients, but also doctors and non-allergic people avoid using chemicals because of concern regarding irritation. Their reluctance to use control agents is probably the biggest obstacle.

The active ingredients of insecticides, such as organophosphates and pyrethroids, have been used as HDM control agents. Although these compounds show some acaricidal efficacy, occasional failure to control domestic mites occurs in practice. This may be due to several of the reasons mentioned above.

Nevertheless, suppression of the HDM population could also inhibit the associated allergens. Several features of various compounds that may be potential control agents have been evaluated. The efficacies of the most expecting compounds are shown here.

Comparison of acaricidal efficacy by the filter paper contact method

The filter paper contact method was used to evaluate the basic acaricidal efficacy of unknown compounds (27). In this experiment, a sheet of filter paper (5 cm × 10 cm) was treated with 500 μL of compound acetone solution at a particular dosage. After drying, the filter paper was folded along the centerline of the long side. Thirty adult mites were released onto the filter paper. The filter paper was then firmly closed with 3 paper clips to prevent the mites from escaping. The test mites were continuously in contact with the treated paper for 24 hours, and mortality was observed under a stereoscopic microscope. By using the mortality rates obtained from each treated plot, the lethal concentration values were calculated by using the probit method.

The acaricidal efficacies of 10 compounds against 3 domestic species, including *D. farinae*, *Tyrophagus putrescentiae* and *Blomia tropicalis*, are summarized in Table 4. *T. putrescentiae* occasionally infests the surface of tatami mats in Japanese residences during the humid season. *B. tropicalis* is distributed in the subtropical regions of Japan and is associated with a medically important allergen similar to *Dermatophagoides* mites. Phenyl salicylate showed superior acaricidal activity against all species of mites, whereas conventional insecticides such as organophosphates and pyrethroids showed lower efficacy except against *B. tropicalis*. Isobornyl thiocyanoacetate (IBTA) demonstrated good efficacy against *D. farinae*; however, it was comparatively less effective against *T. putrescentiae*. Indeed, it is difficult to maintain long-term contact between the mites and the compound residue, and in order to ensure efficiency during practical use, a higher concentration is required. In addition, the efficacy of the compounds occasionally varies depending on the treatment method (28, 29). The suppression effect has at times been evaluated by medium mixing test. Although the mode of action of most acaricides has not been elucidated, one of the reasons for the variation in efficacy seems to be a difference of the intake mechanism in the contact and the medium mixing methods. The control agents should be selected depending on the target species. Moreover, resistance of these domestic mites to acaricides is as yet unknown. In the future, susceptibility of the mites to acaricides should also be evaluated.

Table 4 Acaricidal efficacy of 10 compounds against 3 domestic mite species.

Compound	*LC_{50} values* against each mite species (mg/m^2)*		
	Df	*Tp*	*Bt*
Phenyl Salicylate	9.59	12.2	6.38
IBTA[1)]	15.2	518	63.0
Benzyl Benzoate	23.5	25.3	22.7
S421	43.8	44.9	35.6
Dichlorvos	179	140	9.94
Fenitrothion	261	43.4	8.72
γ -BHC	629	86.3	16.3
PBO[2)]	4,000	>4,000	1,240
Permethrin	>4,000	>4,000	>4,000
pp'-DDT	>4,000	>4,000	>4,000

*: 50% lethal concentration values were calculated by the probit method.

Df: *Dermatophagoides farinae*; Tp: *Tyrophagus putrescentiae*;

Bt: *Blomia tropicalis*

1) Isobornyl thiocyanoacetate, 2) Piperonyl Butoxide

(Data obtained from reference 27)

Ovicidal and development inhibitiory effects of etoxazole

Etoxazole is used against phytophagous mites such as tetranichid mites. This compound has not yet been used against HDMs. It exerts a unique effect on the HDM, in spite of the complete absence of acaricidal efficacy at a concentration of 4,000 mg/m^2, as evaluated by using the contact method (30).

Firstly, the ovicidal efficacies of 4 compounds, namely, etoxazole, IBTA, phenothrin, and pyriproxyfen, were examined using *D. farinae* eggs. Twenty eggs (aged 0–2 days after oviposition) were fixed to a piece of paper sized 20 mm × 20 mm with using a wet brush. Next, 20 μL acetone solution was dripped over the fixed eggs and thenallowed to dry. The hatchability of the eggs was observed 17 days after the treatment. The ovicidal efficacy of the 4 compounds against the *D. farinae* eggs is compared in Table 5. The 50% inhibition concentration (IC_{50}) value of etoxazole was 3.37 ppm, which was about 100 times lower than that of IBTA.

Table 5 Ovicidal activity of 4 compounds against *D. farinae* eggs.

Compound	IC_{50}**ppm*	IC_{90}**ppm*
Etoxazole	3.37	10.2
IBTA	318	2,250
Phenothrin	894	2,010
Pyriproxyfen	4,770	31,000

*:50% and 90% inhibition concentration values were calculated by using the probit method.

(Data obtained from reference 30)

Furthermore, the development inhibition effect of etoxazole against *D. farinae* was observed. Etoxazole was mixed with mite-free medium at a certain dosage. 10 mg of the treated medium was added into a glass vial (14 mm diameter × 33 mm depth). Thirty eggs were fixed to the wall of the vial at a distance from the medium. The vial was sealed by using an impermeable fabric to prevent the hatched mites from escaping. Thirty-two days after the treatment, all the living and dead mites were collected from inside the vial and were classified into the developmental stage: larva, protonymph, tritonymph, male, and female.

Figure 5 shows the proportion of recaptured mites in the 30 eggs that were examined. It was found that most eggs hatched even in the treated plots. It was considered that there was no contact occurred between the eggs did and the treated medium. In the control plot and that treated at 1 ppm concentration , most of the mites that were recaptured were alive and developed into adults. On the other hand, in the plot treated with 16 ppm, more than 40% of the mites were dead and more than 70% of the mites were in the larval stage. Based on this result, it was suggested that etoxazole exerts a growth-regulator like effect against the HDMs.

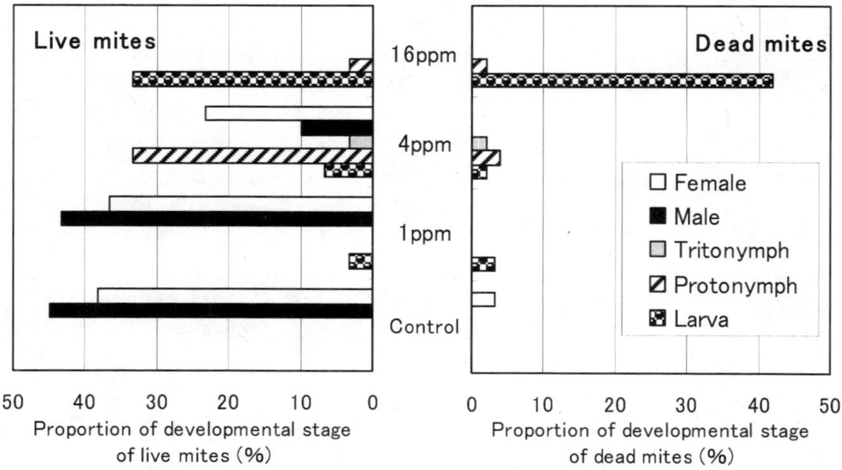

Figure 5 Development inhibition effect of etoxazole against D. farinae obtained at day 32 after treatment.The values indicate the rates of recaptured mites in the examined 30 eggs. (Data obtained from reference 30)

The inhibitory effects of etoxazole against the hatching and molting of *Haemaphysalis longicornis* has also been reported (31). Although more information needs to be accumulated, these unique charecteristics suggest that the use of etoxazole against the HDMs is possible.

Semi-practical efficacy of amidoflumet combined with vacuum cleaning

Amidoflumet is a novel acaricide that was developed by the Sumitomo Chemical Co., Ltd. The LC_{50} value for this compound determined by using the filter paper contact method was 5.42 mg/m^2, which is higher than that of phenyl salicylate (30). Amidoflumet has also been reported to exhibit high acaricidal efficacy against cheyletid mites (32).

In Japan, aerosol sprays, total release aerosols (TRAs), and fumigants are currently available to combat HDMs infestation. The author has evaluated the semi-practical effect of TRAs against *D. farinae* in combination with daily vacuum cleaning (33).

Three pieces of carpet of size 80 cm × 80 cm that harbored mites (≒100 live mites/25 cm^2 [initial value]) were treated with one of the following procedures: (1)The first carpet piece was placed on the living room floor, a TRA was then sprayed on the center of the floor, and the carpet was exposed to the aerosol for 2 hours. After this expousure, the carpet was vacuumed using an electric vacuum cleaner once a week (chemical treatment plot) (2) The 2nd carpet piece was vacuumed once a week without chemical treatment (control A plot) (3) The 3rd carpet had been vacuumed 5 times a week without chemical treatment (control B plot). Each carpet had 16 quadrates with a surface area of 25 cm^2 (Figure 6). These carpets were maintained under stable conditions. During the test period, 10 female adult mites and powdered food were added to each quadrate once a week. Two pieces of the quadrates were cut out from each carpet at every observation point after starting the test. The number of live mites was counted by using the heat escape method (34). The live mites and allergens in the cut carpet pieces were extracted in PBS. These allergens were then quantified by ELISA.

The variations in the mean numbers of live mites and mean quantities of allergen (Der 1) in 2 quadrates are shown in Figure 7. In the chemically treated plot, the number of live mites decreased to 1% of the pretreatment level on day 8. There was no obvious reproduction by day 57. In the control A (weekly vacuuming), no reduction was observed during the test period. In the control B (vacuuming 5 times/week), the apparent decline was delayed until day 43. In the case of Der 1, the amount of the allergen in the chemically treated plot decreased to 45% of the pretreatment level on day 8. However, this reduction was not significant. On the contrary, Der 1 decreased to 8% of the pretreatment level in control B.

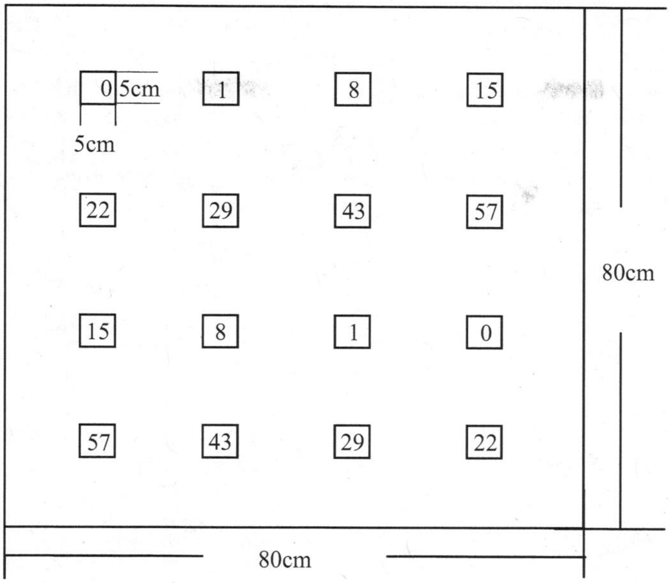

Figure 6 Quadrates in a carpet. The numbers indicate the day after the commencement of the test on which the quadrates were cut.

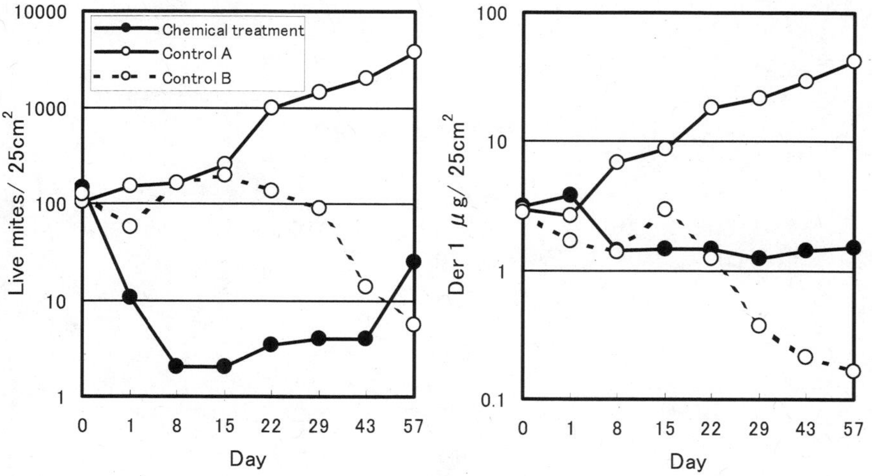

Figure 7 Changes in the numbers of live mites and the quantities of Der 1 after amidoflumet TRA treatment. (Data obtained from reference 33)

Overall, it can be concluded that amidoflumet can rapidly kill live mites. The amidoflumet TRA spray may help people to reduce their daily chores, such as room cleaning and blanket washing. However, vaccuming once aweek cannot be considered effective enough to reduce the levels of the HDM allergen. Hence, in order to achieve the reduction of the allergen in combination with the spray, more frequent vacuuming would be required. Although the practical effects of the chemical agent have to be evaluated under various conditions, we should consider household chemical agents as a complement to daily house maintenance.

Conclusion

HDM allergy is expected to become an important problem in the future considering the increase in the numbers of the allergies in children. In school and home environments, severe mite infestations that exceeding those at thresholds proposed by the Japanese ministries have occassionaly been observed, especially in summer, even on wooden floors that are considered to beeffective for the control of the HDM.

Some effective control agents against HDMs have been developed. The efficacy of some of these compounds sometimes depending on the target mite species, developmental stage, and treatment method. Chemical control measures would reduce daily chores, such as house cleaning or blanket washing. However, chemical treatment should be used as a complement to other environmental strategies to avoid exposure to HDM allergen.

Acknowledgments

The author is grateful to the staff of the Japan Environment Sanitation Center, Mitsuho Yano of Jissen Women's University, and Mitsugu Motoki of Apex Pest Control Co. Ltd. for their cooperation.

References

1. Yamano, Y.; Ishikawa, T.; Nakamura, H.; Moriwaki, Y. *School Health.* **2006**, 48, 325-331 (in Japanese).
2. Sasaki, S. *Allergology.* **1997,** 4, 333-342 (in Japanese).
3. Miyamoto, J.; Ouchi, T. *Sanit. Zool. Entomol.* **1976,** 27, 251-257 (in Japanese).
4. Takaoka, M.; Ishii, A.; Kabasawa, Y.; Ouchi, T. *Sanit. Zool. Entomol.* **1977,** 28, 237-244 (in Japanese).
5. Oshima, S. *Sanit. Zool. Entomol.* **1964,** 15, 233-244 (in Japanese).
6. Yoshikawa, M. *House and Household Insect Pests* **1992,** 14, 88-101 (in Japanese).
7. Konishi, E.; Uehara, K. *Exp. Appl. Acarol.* **1999,** 23, 41-50.
8. Takeda, F.; Toma, T.; Kinjo, N.; Miyagi, I.; Sato, Y. *Med. Entomol. Zool.* **2002,** 53, 163-168.
9. Report of a second international workshop, *J. Allergy Clin. Immunol.* **1992,** 89, 1046-1060.
10. Suto, C.; Sakaki, I.; Itoh, H.; Mitibata, M. *Sanit. Entomol. Zool.* **1993,** 44, 247-255 (in Japanese).
11. Matsumoto, K.; Oakamoto, M.; Wada, Y. *Sanit. Entomol. Zool.* **1986,** 37, 79-90 (in Japanese).
12. Hashimoto, T.; Tanaka, I.; Kamimura, K. *Sanit. Entomol. Zool.* **1993,** 44, 185-195 (in Japanese).
13. Hashimoto, T.; Tajima, F.; Tanaka, I. *J. Acarol. Soc. Jpn.* **1998,** 7, 115-125 (in Japanese).
14. *A guideline for mite control measures in home environments,* The Ministry of Health and Welfare. Japan Environmental Sanitation Center: Kawasaki, JAPAN, **1994**; p147 (in Japanese).
15. Suto, C. *Allergy in Practice* **1997,** 17, 35-40 (in Japanese).
16. *A guideline for mite control measures in home environments – for healeth and confortable life*, The Ministry of Health and Welfare. Gyosei: Tokyo, JAPAN, **1999;** pp 49-56 (in Japanese).
17. *About the disease rate among students in Japanese schools*, URL http://www.mext.go.jp/b_menu/toukei/001/h19.htm
18. *A manual for school environmental hygiene*, The Ministry of Education, Culture, Sports, Science and Technology, Tokyo, JAPAN, **2004**; pp 38-76 (in Japanese).
19. Platts-Mills T.A.E., de Weck A.L., *J. Allergy Clin. Immunol.* **1989**, 83, 416-427.
20. Motoki, M.; Hashimoto, T.; Sasaki, K.; Yoshikawa, A.; Uchida, A. *Med. Entomol. Zool.* **2007,** 58, 275-281 (in Japanese).
21. Hashimoto, T., Tanaka, I. *Pestology* **2006,** 22: 43-48 (in Japanese).
22. Yano, M.; Hashimoto, T.; Muto, A.; Ishii, A. *Med. Entomol. Zool.* **2007,** 58, 199-205 (in Japanese).
23. Hashimoto, T. A report of current status of molds and mite in indoor environments. Center of Housing Renovation and Dispute Settelement Support; Tokyo JAPAN, **2007**; pp 25-43 (in Japanese).

24. Motoki, M. In *Inhalant indoor allergen concerning bronchial asthma.* Koya, N.; Nagakura, T. Eds.; Medical Review. Tokyo, JAPAN, 1999, pp 115-126 (in Japanese).
25. Nishioka, K.; Yasueda, H.; Sairo, H. *J. Allergy Clin. Immunol.* **1998,** 101, 28-32.
26. Haida, M. *Allergology.* **1997,** 4, 343-348 (in Japanese).
27. Hashimoto, T.; Motoyama, N.; Mizutani, K. *Med. Entomol. Zool.* **1999,** 50, 349-354.
28. Mizutani, K. *Bull. Soc. Hyg. Insectic. Sci.*, **1988,** 54, 3-7 (in Japanese).
29. Hirakoso, S. *Pest Control Res.,* **1991,** 6, 19-21 (in Japanese).
30. Hashimoto, T. *Bull. Soc. Hyg. Insectic.* **2004,** 54, 3-7 (in Japanese).
31. Tamura, Y.; Tsubaki, Y.; Terada, Y.; Kohmoto, M.; Kamio, T. *Med. Entomol. Zool.* **2004,** 55, 303-311.
32. Mori, T.;Takada, Y.; Hatakoshi, M.; Matsuo, N. *Biosci. Biotechnol. Biochem.* **2004,** 68, 425-427.
33. Hashimoto, T.; Minagawa, K.; Koizumi, T.; Kamezaki, H.; Takita, K. *Med. Entomol. Zool.* **2004,** 55, 47-53 (in Japanese).
34. Vargas, M. *Internat. J. Acarol.* **2002,** 28, 277-278.

Novel Approaches and Resistance Management

Chapter 9

Controlling Dengue Virus Transmission in the Field with Genetically Modified Mosquitoes

Ken E. Olson and Alexander W. E. Franz

Arthropod-borne and Infectious Diseases Laboratory (AIDL), Department of Microbiology, Immunology & Pathology, Colorado State University, Fort Collins, CO 80523

The mosquito-borne dengue viruses pose significant threats to public health. Transgenesis technology has been developed for *Aedes aegypti*, the major vector of dengue viruses, to better understand vector competence and negatively impact virus transmission. Integration of exogenous DNA into the germline is achieved with class II transposable elements (TEs). Marker genes expressing fluorescing proteins are used to monitor the insertion of these elements. Endogenous promoters are available to express effector genes in tissues relevant to infection by mosquito-borne viruses. Proof-of-concept experiments show that expression of anti-viral genes can have a profound impact on transmission. A major hurdle to overcome is development of efficient genetic drive systems that spread effector genes into local vector populations. We have developed RNA interference (RNAi)-based transgenic resistance against dengue virus type 2 (DENV2) in *Ae. aegypti*. The idea is to boost the innate antiviral RNAi response in the mosquito as infection is occurring. An intron-containing inverted-repeat cDNA derived from the prM coding region of DENV2 RNA has been inserted into the *Mariner Mos1* TE. The bloodmeal inducible, midgut specific carboxypeptidase A promoter transcribes the effector gene. A mosquito line (Carb77) has been generated having a single copy of the transgene expressing the inverted-repeat RNA in the midgut. Carb77 mosquitoes are highly resistant to challenge with DENV2. Resistance to DENV2 is reversible by impairing the RNAi pathway. An assessment of Carb77 mosquitoes' potential to introgress into wild type strains, and the development of transgenic mosquitoes having resistance to all four DENV serotypes is discussed.

Dengue Viruses and their Principal Mosquito Vector, *Aedes aegypti*

Dengue viruses (DENV) are considered to be the most important mosquito borne arboviruses infecting humans (*1*). The viruses are endemic in about 100 countries and they infect annually an estimated 50 million people worldwide (*2, 3*). The outcome of the disease can vary dramatically ranging from no symptoms or slight febrile illness to severe hemorrhagic manifestations (dengue hemorrhagic fever, DHS) or dengue shock syndrome (DSS). The latter manifestation means circulatory collapse as a consequence of severe hemorrhagic fever. DHS and DSS are more typical for children that became infected with DENV and for DSS the case fatality rate can reach ~5% (*4*). The molecular and immunological mechanisms that cause these varying disease outcomes of DENV infections are only now being elucidated (*5*). Currently, there are no therapeutics or safe vaccines against the virus, prompting the research community to search for ways to interrupt the DENV disease cycle by tackling the mosquito vector (*6*). Mosquito control programs were very efficient between 1950-1970 in the Americas to suppress mosquito populations in urban areas (*7*). Systematic insecticide spraying campaigns diminished *Ae. aegypti* populations in South and Central America, leading to only rare occurrences of DENV epidemics (*7*). During the past 30 years however, insecticide applications became more erratic causing a severe surge of *Ae. aegypti* populations throughout Latin America. In addition, resistance to certain insecticides such as Temophos and Cypermethrin has become apparent among populations of this mosquito species (*8, 9*). As a novel, alternative approach we have been investigating whether genetic modification of *Ae. aegypti* is a feasible approach to reduce the mosquito's vector competence for DENV in the field leading to a decline in virus prevalence.

DENV are spherical enveloped RNA viruses belonging to the Flaviviridae (genus: *Flavivirus*) (*10, 11, 12*). They are separated into four distinct serotypes (= species), dengue virus 1-4 (DENV1-4), which all have common overall morphologies and vector interactions but vary considerably in their genome sequences as well as antigenic regions. The single stranded positive sense RNA genome (~11,000 nt) of DENV is enclosed in a nucleocapsid which is surrounded by a phospholipid bilayer containing a glycosylated envelope protein and a non-glycosilated membrane protein. The gene order (5' to 3' of the RNA genome) is: C (capsid), prM (pre-Membrane), E (envelope), NS1, NS2A, NS2B, NS3, NS4A, NS4B, NS5 (non-structural proteins). The DENV RNA genome encodes a single polyprotein that is cleaved co- and post-translationally by viral proteases and host signalases into multi-functional protein units. During replication of the viral RNA the virus forms a transient dsRNA intermediate which is a potential trigger of the host's innate RNAi mechanism.

Viruses causing epidemic dengue disease are transmitted in nature by *Ae. aegypti*. This mosquito species is highly anthropophilic and has been shown to be the main vector during severe DENV outbreaks in urban areas (*7*). The vector becomes persistently infected with DENV (*13*). After ingesting a viremic bloodmeal, the mosquito midgut epithelium is the first tissue that becomes infected with the virus (*14*). About six to seven days later the virus starts to disseminate in *Ae. aegypti* from the midgut to secondary tissues such as fat body, nerve tissue, hemocytes and eventually the salivary glands (*15, 16*). Once the latter are infected the mosquito is able to transmit the virus to new hosts. The extrinsic incubation period (EIP) for DENV in *Ae. aegypti* is 12-14 days under laboratory conditions. The vector competence of certain populations can vary considerably for different DENV strains (*17*). This could be attributed to differences in the mosquito's efficiency to elicit innate immune responses against the virus. The midgut appears to be a major organ that determines vector competence for DENV in *Ae. aegypti* (*18*). Midgut infection (MIB) and midgut escape barriers (MEB) described for DENV are highly dependent on the particular vector strain / virus strain combinations (*17, 19, 20*). In presence of a MIB, the virus is not able to efficiently infect the midgut epithelium. In presence of a MEB, the virus readily infects the midgut epithelium but its dissemination to secondary tissues is inhibited. The MEB for arboviruses has been suggested to be influenced by the mosquito's innate RNAi pathway (*21, 22*).

The RNA Interference Pathway in Drosophila and Mosquitoes

Drosophila has been shown to have RNAi as an antiviral defense pathway (*23, 24, 25.*). Our group at AIDL has investigated over the past 10 years whether mosquitoes also possess a similar cellular RNAi mechanism which can affect arbovirus infections. In eukaryotes, the RNAi pathway can be divided into four discrete biochemical steps: (i) dsRNA processing, (ii) maintenance of siRNA 5' phosphate termini to facilitate RNA Induced Silencing Complex (RISC) incorporation, (iii) small interfering RNA (siRNA) loading into RISC, (iv) siRNA-based degradation of target mRNA (*26*). In Drosophila, two genes encoding enzymes with RNAse III-like nuclease activity have been identified, *dcr1* and *dcr2* (*26*). Both act in two distinct RNA silencing pathways. Whereas dicer-1 is responsible for the processing of microRNAs (miRNAs) in the miRNA silencing pathway, dicer-2 is the enzyme of the siRNA silencing pathway that processes dsRNA into small 22 nt siRNA duplexes. Dicer-2 is tightly associated with an auxillary dsRNA binding protein named R2D2 to efficiently bind siRNA duplexes (*27*). According to a recent model the siRNA duplex containing dicer-2/R2D2 complex is incorporated into RISC whose major enzymatic component is argonaute-2 (*28*). The passenger strand of the siRNA duplex is cleaved from the guide strand which interacts with argonaute-2 and guides the latter to target mRNA containing the complementary sequence. (*29, 30*). After hybridization argonaute-2 cleaves the phosphodiester backbone of the target mRNA, thus silencing specifically recognized RNA.

We identified orthologs of the RNAi pathway genes *dcr1*, *dcr2*, *r2d2*, and *ago2* among the genomes of *Anopheles gambiae* and *Ae. aegypti* (*22, 31, 32*). Several research teams demonstrated in functional assays that *dcr2*, *r2d2*, and *ago2* are essential components of the siRNAi pathway in *An. gambiae* and *Ae. aegypti (22, 31, 32, 33).* In either mosquito species the siRNAi pathway was compromised after transient silencing of *dcr2, r2d2*, or *ago2* through intrathoracic injection of gene-specific dsRNAs (*22, 31, 34*). As a consequence orally acquired DENV2, Sindbis virus (SINV, Togaviridae) or O'nyong-nyong virus (ONNV, Togaviridae; transmitted by *An. gambiae*) replicated in those mosquitoes much more efficiently, reaching significantly higher titers as compared to non-compromised controls. Furthermore, as shown for DENV2 the EIP was up to three days shorter in immune compromised *Ae. aegypti* as compared to controls (*34*). These findings indicate that replication of different arboviruses such as SINV, ONNV, or DENV2 in mosquitoes is kept in check by their innate RNAi pathway. Nevertheless, all these viruses are capable of persistently infecting their mosquito hosts leading to virus transmission.

In a number of experimental approaches we demonstrated that – as in Drosophila (*23, 24, 25*) – the mosquito RNAi machinery functions as an antiviral immunity mechanism. Arboviruses such as DENV, are targets for RNAi in adult mosquitoes (*34, 35*). Furthermore, Xi *et al.* (*36*) discovered that after infection with DENV2 *Ae. aegypti* activates also other innate immune responses which are mainly controlled by the Toll pathway. We showed that transient silencing of ONNV by intrathoracic injection of dsRNA derived from the nsP3 region of the virus profoundly inhibited viral replication in the mosquito (*31*). Similar results were obtained for SINV following the same experimental approach. When inserting a cDNA fragment derived from the prM encoding region of DENV2 into a recombinant SINV strain and injecting this modified virus into female mosquitoes they became refractory to orally acquired DENV2 (*37*). Further analysis showed that systemic expression of short DENV2 derived sequences by a recombinant SINV strongly triggered the RNAi pathway against DENV2. In C6/36 *Ae. albopictus* cells we eventually demonstrated that stably transformed cells which transcribed inverted-repeat (IR) RNAs containing DENV2 derived sequences were completely resistant to the virus (*38*). This observation encouraged us to follow the same principle when designing anti-DENV effector genes for the generation of transgenic mosquitoes to be refractory to the virus.

Germline Transformation of *Aedes aegypti*

Principle

The methodology of mosquito transgenesis is largely derived from extensive experimentation with Drosophila (*39*). Until now mosquitoes of three different genera, *Culex, Aedes*, and *Anopheles* have been genetically transformed for laboratory studies (*40, 41, 42, 43, 44*). The protocol we used for germline transformation of *Ae. aegypti* was based on that described by Jasinskiene *et al.* (*43*). The basic genetic components that are required for mosquito germline transformation are:

- Transposable element (TE) as insertion vector
- Selection marker
- Gene-of-interest expression cassette
- Transposase source

Until now four different Class II TEs have been used for the germline transformation of insects: *Mariner* (*Mos1*), *piggyBac*, *Hermes*, and *Minos* originally isolated from *Drosophila mauritiana*, the cabbage looper *Trichoplusia ni*, the house fly *Musca domestica*, and *Drosophila hydei*, respectively (*43, 45, 46, 47*). In mosquitoes any of these TEs demonstrated only very low mobility (*48*). For our experiments we chose the non-autonomous mariner *Mos1* TE in which the transposase was disrupted by a fluorescent selection marker such as Enhanced Green Fluorescent Protein (EGFP) under control of the synthetic, eye and nerve tissue specific *3xP3* promoter (*49*). The gene of interest was inserted next to the selection marker expression cassette between the right and left arms of the TE. This so-called donor plasmid was co-injected together with a helper plasmid encoding the open reading frame (ORF) of the *Mariner* transposase under control of a heat shock promoter into preblastoderm embryos of *Ae. aegypti*. As recipient strain we used an eye pigment deficient mutant of RexD originating from Puerto Rico, Higg's White Eye (HWE) (*50*). It appeared to be critically important to use mosquitoes lacking eye pigmentation as recipients for germline transformations because only in those fluorescent markers such as EGFP, DsRed or Enhanced Cyan Fluorescent Protein (ECFP) are easily visible under a fluorescent microscope. After micro-injection into germline tissue expression of the transposase facilitated integration of the modified TE into the host DNA. Since both, transposase and donor DNA were not physically linked to each other the TE lost its transposase source after integration into the host DNA and thus could not be re-mobilized in subsequent generations of the transformed mosquito line. This allowed stable gene-of-interest expression levels throughout many generations of the line.

Using Transgenic Mosquitoes for Two Different Strategies: Population Replacement or Population Reduction

Transgenic mosquito technology can be used to pursue two major strategies, population replacement and population reduction. The experimental work conducted by our work group and outlined in this chapter aims at population replacement, i.e. replacing DENV competent mosquitoes for genetically engineered ones that are not competent for the virus. In this paragraph, we would like to give a brief overview on strategies for insect population reduction.

The insect population reduction strategy that has been used in the field until now is Sterile Insect Technology (SIT). It has been successfully implemented to reduce and/or eliminate populations of the New Word screw worm fly (*Cochliomyia hominivorax*), the Mediterranean fruit fly (*Ceratitis capitata*), and the codling moth (*Cydia pomonella*) from various countries of the Americas (*51, 52*). This 'classical' procedure does not involve the production of transgenic insects. Instead males of the target insect are selected and sterilized by irradiation in rearing facilities where the females are eliminated. Over a prolonged period of time these sterile males are released in vast numbers in areas where target insect populations are present. If the procedure is successful most of the females of the target populations will choose the more abundant sterile males as mating partners and consequently not produce any offspring. Eventually the population will collapse. This approach is very labor intense, costly and bears the risk of producing sterile males with reduced fitness that are not able to outcompete wild type males in the field. A promising improvement of this strategy, designated Release of Insects carrying a Dominant Lethal (RIDL) involves the genetic engineering of insects that carry a dominant female-specific lethal trait that is repressible for rearing purposes. In presence of a chemical food additive such as tetracyclin males and females both are viable. In absence of tetracyclin however, only males are viable and fertile whereas females die. Following release of these engineered insects and mating with wild types all of their progeny would be heterozygous for the dominant trait. Since tetracyclin is absent in the field females will eventually vanish from the population within a few generations causing it to collapse. The molecular mechanism underlying RIDL has been well described (*51, 52*). In a recent effort this system has been adapted for the population reduction of *Ae. aegypti* and shown to be functional under laboratory conditions (*53*).

Genes-of-Interest

Promoters

To allow proper spatial and temporal expression of effector genes in *Ae. aegypti* the availability of suitable promoters is critically important. In earlier experiments we tried to use the constitutive *poly-ubiquitin* promoter from Drosophila or the baculovirus *ie1* promoter to drive marker gene expression in transgenic mosquitoes (*54, 55*). None of these attempts resulted in predictable gene-of-interest expression levels thus prompting us to focus on promoters originating from genes of *Ae. aegypti* instead. Indeed, several *Ae. aegypti* promoters have been isolated and tested for transgene expression levels by various research groups. Among those were the midgut-specific carboxypeptidase A *(AeCPA)*, ferritin heavy-chain homologue (*HCH*), and glutamine synthetase (*GS*), the fat body-specific vitellogenin 1 (*Vg*), as well as the salivary gland-specific apyrase (*Apy*) and maltase-like 1 (*Mal1*), respectively (*56, 57, 58, 59, 60, 61, 62, 63*). *Apy* and *Mal1* appeared to allow only weak expression levels in salivary glands of transformed *Ae. aegypti*. The *HCH*, *GS*, and *Vg* promoters have been analyzed in functional assays based on cell culture systems (*57, 62, 64*). However, in transgenic mosquitoes only the latter of those was able to drive heterologous gene expression in an inducible, tissue-specific manner. The vitellogenin 1 gene encodes the major yolk protein precursor of *Ae. aegypti* and is up-regulated to high levels in the female fat body, reaching a peak at ~24 h after receiving of a bloodmeal. Of the midgut-specific promoters isolated so far only the 1122 bp *AeCPA* caused strong transgene expression levels in mosquitoes (*60*, *61*). We confirmed this by generating transgenic mosquitoes that expressed EGFP under the control of the *AeCPA* promoter. In two lines, Carb/gfp52 and Carb/gfp105 EGFP expression was very strong, encompassing the entire midgut epithelium at 24 h to 72 h post bloodmeal (pbm). See Figure 1.

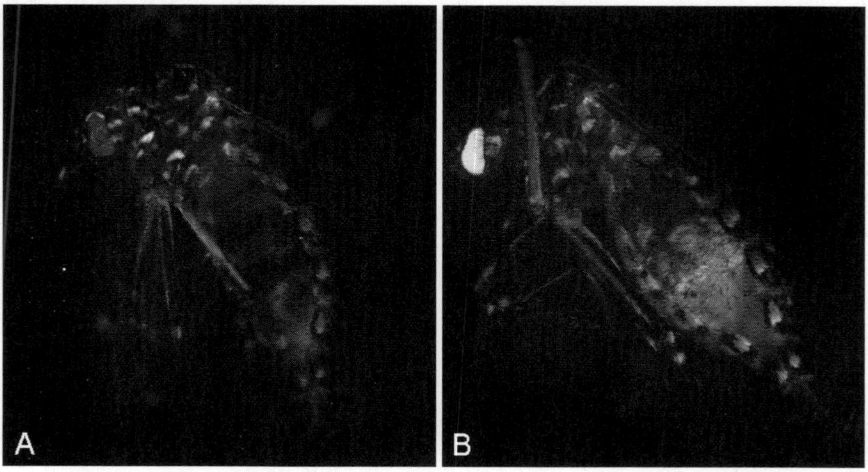

Figure 1. Bloodmeal inducible, midgut specific expression profile of the AeCPA promoter in transgenic Ae. aegypti of family Carb/gfp105. Mosquitoes were viewed under a fluorescent microscope equipped with EGFP specific filters. (A) Bloodfed female of the HWE recipient strain. (B) Carb/gfp105 at 24 h post bloodmeal. Eye specific EGFP expression originated from the 3xP3 promoter driven selection marker of the Mariner Mos1 transposable element.

However, in line Carb/gfp112 midgut specific marker gene expression was always very weak throughout the time course and in another nine lines there was no EGFP expression at all in bloodfed females. This indicated a strong influence of position effects on transgene expression levels since transgene integration sites differed in all these lines. The *AeCPA* gene encodes an exopeptidase that is expressed in the midgut epithelium of female *Ae. aegypti* to proteolytically cleave polypeptides from proteins acquired along with the bloodmeal inside the midgut lumen. Expression of the gene is strongly up-regulated between 4h and 36h after receiving of a bloodmeal. Because the midgut is the first organ of the mosquito which becomes infected with DENV, we anticipated that the midgut epithelium would be an ideal tissue to express anti-DENV effectors. Furthermore, effector gene expression at the very beginning of bloodmeal digestion would tackle the incoming virus when it is in its most vulnerable state: at the on-set of *de novo* synthesis in midgut tissue before being able to establish strong foci of infection.

Eventually, we chose the *AeCPA* and *Vg* promoters to generate transgenic mosquitoes that target DENV by triggering the RNAi pathway against the virus.

Anti-DENV Effectors

Our aim was to generate anti-DENV effector genes that would trigger the mosquito's innate RNAi pathway to target and destroy the viral RNA in a homology dependent manner. The principle design of such anti-DENV effectors was based on inverted-repeat (IR) DNAs which contained a few hundred nucleotide (nt) cDNA fragment derived from the DENV genome in sense and anti-sense orientations. The sense and antisense cDNA fragments were separated by the small 64 nt intron of the salivary gland specific *Ae. aegypti* sialokinin I gene (*65*). As reported by several authors (*66, 67*) the incorporation of a small functional intron appeared to enhance the formation of a perfect dsRNA structure upon transcription of the IR DNA, acting as the trigger for the RNAi cascade in the cell. To target DENV2 we chose in earlier experiments a 291 nt cDNA derived from the prM region of the DENV2 (Jamaica 1409) genome. In cell culture experiments and in transient silencing experiments using mosquitoes, this cDNA fragment caused sufficient silencing of DENV2 (*37, 38*). Considering higher target specificity when using slightly larger fragment sizes we eventually chose a 578 nt cDNA fragment of a similar region of the DENV2 genome as the effector gene in several transgenic mosquito lines described below.

The promising results we obtained when using IR DNA constructs that targeted DENV2 in mosquitoes encouraged us to design a tetravalent effector gene that would tackle all four serotypes of the virus simultaneously. In an initial attempt we were focusing on the 3'UTR region of the viral RNA which contained a 146 nt stretch with >90% similarity among all four DENV serotypes. In a transient assay, we intrathoracically injected mosquitoes with dsRNA derived from this region of the viral RNA before exposing them to an artificial bloodmeal containing any of the four DENV serotypes. However, virus titers never appeared to be depleted in these mosquitoes as compared to mock-injected controls suggesting that the 3'UTR of DENVs is not strongly targeted by the RNAi machinery. Therefore we decided to generate a tetravalent effector gene containing short cDNA fragments derived from all four DENV serotypes that were fused together as a 'hybrid' molecule. In this approach we chose the NS5 gene of the virus as a target region. Genome alignments of several strains of all four virus serotypes revealed that NS5, encoding the viral polymerase, is the most conserved gene of the virus. For each DENV serotype we generated nine sets of dsRNA, each about 300 nt in size that altogether spanned the entire region of the 2700 nt NS5 gene. In transient assays we intrathoracically injected the dsRNA into mosquitoes three days before challenging them with the respective virus serotype. When virus titers were analyzed in those mosquitoes at seven or 12 days post infectious bloodmeal (pibm) it became obvious that certain dsRNA fragments derived from certain DENV serotypes caused higher RNA silencing efficiencies than others. Based on the results of this experiment we chose NS5 fragment #8 of DENV2, #7 of DENV1, #6 of DENV4, and #5 of DENV3 to assemble the hybrid molecule in that order using fusion PCR techniques. The resulting 1167 nt fragment was inserted into the IR DNA expression plasmid in sense and anti-sense orientations and separated by the small intron of the sialokinin I gene. Currently we are generating transgenic mosquitoes in which the tetravalent IR DNA is under control of the *AeCPA* promoter.

Transgenic Mosquito Lines Developed to Block DENV Replication

Vg28, Vg29, Vg40

We co-injected the *Mariner Mos1* helper plasmid and the modified *Mos1* donor plasmid containing the 578 nt IR DNA derived from DENV2 under control of the 2100 nt *Vg* promoter into 1440 embryos of *Ae. aegypti*. Out of those 73 larvae survived and 46 G_0 families were established after outcrossing to HWE mosquitoes. Among three families, Vg28, Vg29, and Vg40 we found larvae expressing EGFP in their eyes. We maintained these three transgenic lines for further analysis. In Northern analysis we revealed relatively weak transgene expression levels in the fat body of Vg28 at 6-30 h pbm, intermediate expression in that of Vg29 at 6-24 h pbm, and relatively strong expression in that of Vg40 at 10-24 h pbm. These slightly different transgene expression profiles could be attributed to position effects. We decided to challenge Vg40 with a DENV2 containing bloodmeal to evaluate if silencing the virus in the fat body of mosquitoes would be sufficient to block infection of other secondary tissues such as salivary glands, eventually inhibiting transmission of the virus. A major challenge of this experimental approach was the fact that the *Vg* promoter drives gene expression levels only for a time period of ~24 h pbm in fat body tissue whereas DENV2 requires a minimum time period of 5-7 days pibm to disseminate from the midgut and establish infection foci in the fat body. Thus we needed to give Vg40 mosquitoes two consecutive bloodmeals, the first one containing DENV2, the second one which was given five days later did not contain virus. Twenty four h, 48 h, and 72 h after the second bloodmeal females were analyzed for virus titers by plaque assays. None of these experiments indicated any levels of resistance of Vg40 mosquitoes to DENV2 since titers of those were very similar to the HWE control. Similar results were obtained when we first gave Vg40 mosquitoes a virus-free bloodmeal followed by intrathoracic injection of DENV2. Salivary glands of Vg40 mosquitoes and HWE both showed strong presence of viral antigen at 4 days post injection when analyzed by IFA.

Thus, we considered the expression of an RNAi trigger against DENV2 in fat body tissue of *Ae. aegypti* not sufficient to significantly reduce the mosquito's vector competence for the virus.

Carb77

A total of 1160 preblastoderm embryos of the *Ae. aegypti* HWE strain were co-injected with the *Mariner Mos1* helper plasmid and the *Mos1* derived donor plasmid containing the 578 nt IR DNA targeting DENV2 under control of the *AeCPA* promoter (*32*). See Figure 2. We established 91 G_0 families from the surviving embryos and eventually selected one family, Carb77 that displayed strong EGFP expression in eyes of larvae, pupae, and adults. After outcrossing to the HWE recipient strain followed by intercrossing of transgenic phenotypes we analyzed mosquitoes of this line for their transgenic genotype, gene-of-interest expression levels as well as resistance to DENV2. Southern blot data suggested that there were only one transgene integration event in Carb77 mosquitoes. Using genome-walking we could identify the physical integration site within the mosquito's genome. It is located within a non-coding region of a non-repetitive sequence motif belonging to supercontig 1.278 (VectorBase) (A.WE. Franz *et al., unpublished*). A single transgene integration event within a non-coding region of the genome is considered a 'preferred situation' to ensure stable transgene heritability, transgene expression levels and robust fitness of the transgenic organism.

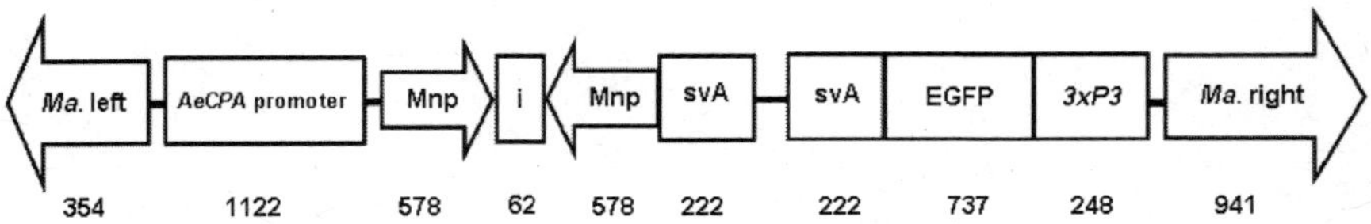

Figure 2. Schematic representation of the Carb77 transgene based on a modified Mariner Mos1 transposable element containing the eye-specific fluorescent selection marker cassette and the 578 nt IR DNA targeting DENV2 under control of the AeCPA promoter. Abbreviations: Ma. left, Ma. right = left, right arm of Mariner Mos1; Mnp = cDNAs of the DENV2 prM encoding region in sense and antisense orientations, respectively; i = minor intron of the Ae. aegypti sialokinin I gene; svA = polyadenylation signal of Simian virus 40 VP1 gene. Numbers below indicate the sizes of the DNA fragments in base pairs. (Reproduced from reference 32. Copyright 2006 National Academy of Sciences of the USA.)

Northern analysis revealed that the anti-DENV2 effector was expressed in midgut tissue of Carb77 females that had received a bloodmeal 27 and 48 h before. See Figure 3. IR RNA transcripts were not detected in those females that were not bloodfed or in tissues other than the midgut. In a ribonuclease protection assay we revealed that the IR DNA was recognized and processed by the mosquito's RNAi machinery. We were able to detect small interfering (si)RNAs derived from the effector among total RNA extracted from females, at 1 day pbm. Carb77 females were refractory to DENV2 as compared to the highly susceptible HWE recipient. We were able to demonstrate this by different analytical approaches. Using immunofluorescence assays (IFA) viral antigen was not detectable in most of the midguts of Carb77 females that had received a DENV2 containing bloodmeal seven days before. In those midguts in which viral antigen was detectable the infection foci were very localized and small as compared to the HWE control where foci often encompassed most of the epithelium. This indicated that in Carb77 females the interference with DENV2 replication occurred in midgut tissue as anticipated by the expression profile of the effector gene. Consequently, we expected to see no or only very inefficient dissemination of viral antigen from midguts of Carb77 mosquitoes to secondary tissues such as salivary glands. Indeed, when analyzing salivary gland tissue of Carb77 at 22 days pibm by IFA, DENV2 envelope antigen was not detectable whereas almost all of the HWE salivary glands showed strong presence of viral antigen. Curiously, the fat body tissue surrounding the salivary glands of Carb77 mosquitoes occasionally appeared to be virus infected.

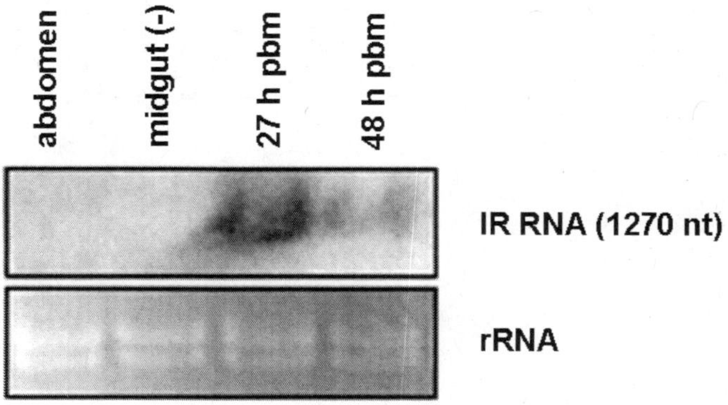

Figure 3. Expression of the anti-DENV2 effector in bloodfed Carb77 females. Total RNAs extracted from midguts or carcasses of Carb77 females at 27h and 48h post bloodmeal or after a sugarmeal (-) were tested by Northern analysis. Membranes were hybridized with a radio-isotope labeled RNA probe corresponding to the anti-DENV2 effector. Ribosomal RNAs are shown in the lower panel to indicate amounts of RNA loaded per lane. (Reproduced from reference 32. Copyright 2006 National Academy of Sciences of the USA.)

When DENV2 was intrathoracically injected into Carb77 mosquitoes, thus by-passing the replication barrier in the midgut epithelium salivary gland tissue became infected with the virus to levels similar of the HWE control. Northern analysis supported the observation that in Carb77 mosquitoes viral replication was inhibited in midgut tissue. See Figure 4 A. After 2 days pibm, viral RNA was not detectable among total RNA extracted from midgut tissue for a time period of 14 days. In the HWE control, viral RNA was strongly present for a time period of up to 10 days pibm with the exception of day 3 which apparently represented the eclipse phase for the virus. Thus, the viral RNA detected before day 3 most likely originated from the virus added to the artificial bloodmeal. When we compared DENV2 titers in Carb77 females with those in HWE at 7, 10, 14 days pibm virus titers in the former were consistently lower than in the latter. See Figure 4 B. During the entire time course of 7-14 days only 2/69 transgenic mosquitoes exceeded titers of 2000 plaque forming units (pfu)/ml whereas more than 50% of the HWE developed titers above 2500 pfu/ml. Obviously, the most relevant criterion when assessing levels of refractoriness is the amount of virus that could be potentially transmitted by a mosquito vector to a mammalian host. However, for DENV there is no small animal model readily available that would allow us to test for that *in vivo*. Therefore, we developed an *in vitro* transmission assay in which mosquitoes probed at 14 days pibm on a salt containing solution that was placed between two Parafilm membranes. Feeding solutions and mosquitoes were then analyzed by plaque assays for the presence of infectious DENV2.

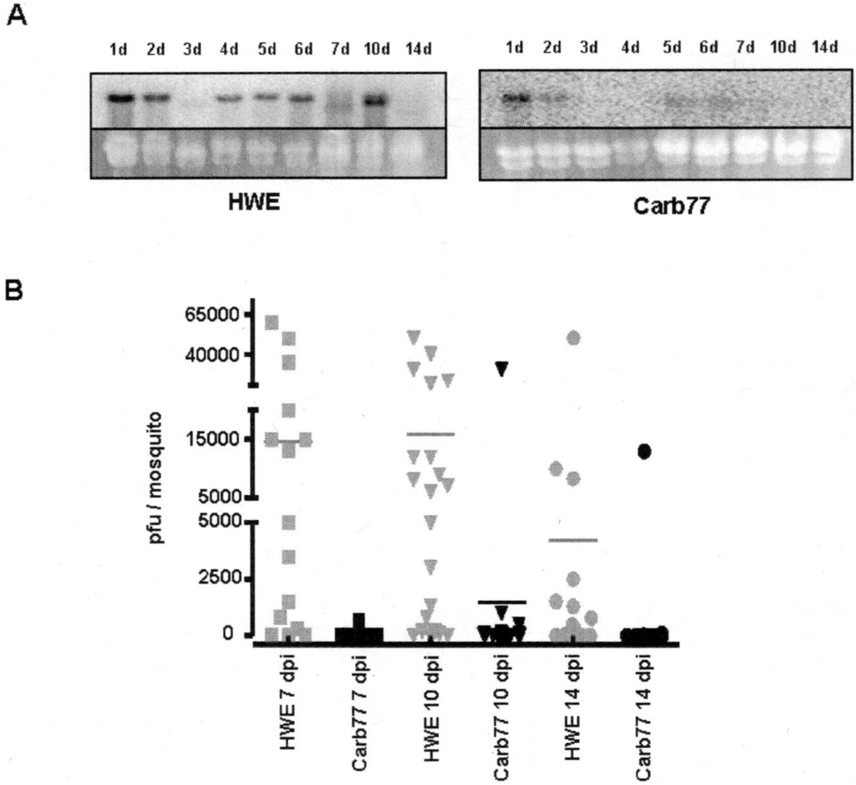

Figure 4. Confirmation of the resistance phenotype of Carb77 mosquitoes by Northern analysis and plaque assays. (A) After receiving a DENV2 containing bloodmeal total RNAs were extracted from midguts of HWE (left blot) and Carb77 females (right blot) and tested by Northern analysis for the presence of viral RNA at 1-14 days post infection. Ribosomal RNAs are shown below as loading controls. (B) At 7, 10, 14 days following a DENV2 containing bloodmeal (dpi) individual HWE and Carb77 females were analyzed for the presence of infectious virus by plaque assays using LLC-MK2 monkey kidney cells. (Reproduced from reference 32. Copyright 2006 National Academy of Sciences of the USA.)

Two out of three feeding solutions each on which 15 females of Carb77 mosquito had probed before had no virus titers and the titer of the remaining one, $1x10^5$ pfu/ml, was about 2-fold lower than the average titer of the three solutions on which HWE had probed. See Figure 5.

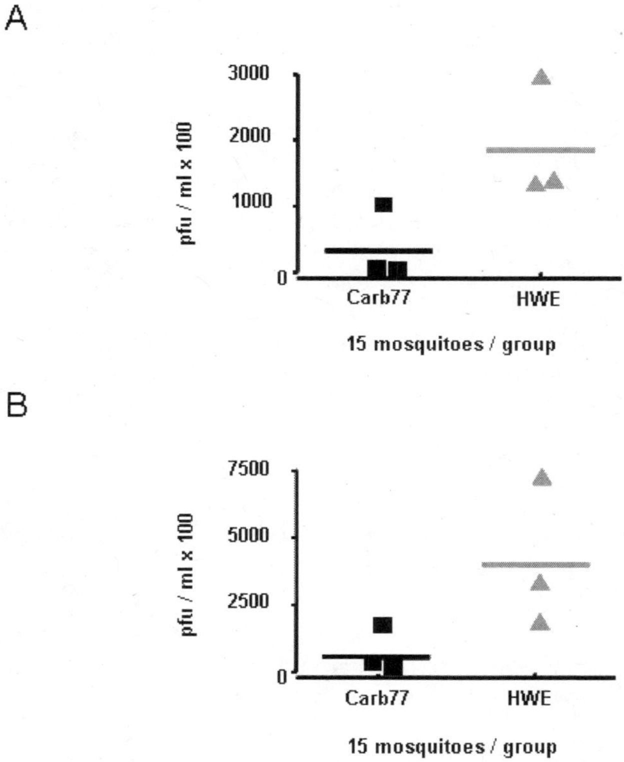

Figure 5. Transmission potential of Carb77 and HWE females for DENV2 at 14 days post infectious bloodmeal. Three groups of 15 DENV2 infected females each were allowed to probe and feed for 1h on a salt containing feeding solution that was placed between two Parafilm membranes stretched over a glass feeder. After probing feeding solutions (A) and mosquitoes (B) were collected and subjected to plaque assays using LLC-MK2 monkey kidney cells. (Reproduced from reference 32. Copyright 2006 National Academy of Sciences of the USA.)

This suggests that the DENV2 transmission potential was severely diminished and often completely lost among Carb77 mosquitoes. We confirmed that the resistance phenotype of Carb77 was homology dependent since only DENV2 replication and transmission was blocked in these mosquitoes but not that of other DENV serotypes such as DENV4 (Philippines H241). Indeed, DENV4 infected Carb77 mosquitoes to an extent that was very similar to the HWE control. This finding prompted us to assess how stringent the phenomenon of homology dependence was by challenging Carb77 mosquitoes with DENV2 strains other than Jamaica 1409 the effector was derived from. Carb77 mosquitoes that were challenged with DENV2 Indonesia 1051 or Puerto-Rico 159 representing the Cosmopolitan and American genotypes of the virus, respectively showed levels of refractoriness that were similar to that when challenged with the Jamaica 1409 strain of the American-Asian genotype (A.W.E. Franz *et al.*, *unpublished*). In a further test we wanted to confirm that the DENV2 resistance phenotype of Carb77 was based on triggering the RNAi pathway against the virus. Therefore we transiently silenced components of the RNAi pathway in Carb77 mosquitoes around three days before they were challenged with a DENV2 containing bloodmeal. To silence RNAi pathway genes mosquitoes were intrathoracically injected each with 500 ng of ~500 bp dsRNAs targeting the *Ae. aegypti* gene orthologs of *ago2*, *r2d2*, or *dcr2*. Carb77 mosquitoes whose RNAi pathway was transiently compromised completely lost their resistance phenotype for the virus, as shown by an up to 20-fold increase of virus titers in these as compared to mock injected controls (A.W.E. Franz *et al.*, *unpublished*).

In summary, the generation and thorough analysis of Carb77 mosquitoes showed us that - as a proof of principle - it is feasible to design and produce transgenic *Ae. aegypti* which are refractory to arboviruses such as DENV2 under controlled laboratory conditions.

Outlook: Using DENV Refractory Mosquitoes for Population Replacement in the Field

Genetically modified mosquitoes to be refractory to DENV must fulfill several critically important requirements before becoming applicable for mosquito population replacement strategies in the field:

- They need to be engineered to be refractory to all four serotypes of DENV.
- Their resistance phenotype has to be stably maintained after introgression of their anti-DENV effector into a wild type population.
- Their overall fitness has to be similar to that of the wild types in the target population to avoid strong selection against the genetically modified mosquitoes.
- The inheritance pattern of their transgene has to be stable and species-specific to rule out horizontal gene transfer to non-target insect populations.

Currently, we are generating transgenic *Ae. aegypti* to be refractory to all four serotypes of DENV. Furthermore, we are testing whether the resistance phenotype of Carb77 is maintained after this line had been back-crossed for multiple generations to a Genetically Diverse Laboratory Strain (GDLS). The GDLS was generated as a hybrid of 10 *Ae. aegypti* populations collected two years ago from different DENV endemic areas of the south-western part of Mexico. Eventually we will compare the fitness of GDLS x Carb77 hybrids to that of GDLS.

In the field a relatively slight fitness loss of the transgenic hybrid could be compensated for by the use of a powerful gene drive system which would be tightly linked to the anti-DENV effector. Gene drive systems are supposed to fix genes in populations at a faster rate than would be expected when inherited in a Mendelian manner (*68*). Several gene drive systems have been proposed for insects: autonomous TE, underdominance, meiotic drive, *Wolbachia*, homing endonuclease, Maternal Effect Dominant Embryonic Arrest (Medea) (*69, 70, 71, 72, 73, 74, 75, 76, 77, 78, 79, 80, 81, 82*). Whereas in Drosophila, the *P*-element has been shown to be extremely mobile it failed to mobilize in mosquitoes (*39*). Likewise, any of the four TEs described above showed only very limited mobility in *Ae. aegypti (48)*. Thus, using autonomous TEs as potent gene drivers in mosquitoes is currently not considered to be a feasible strategy. Meiotic drive has been described in *Culex* sp. as well as *Ae. aegypti* (*71, 72, 73*). In this system one or several genes on the male sex determination locus distort the maturation of gametes which contain sensitive response alleles on the female sex determination locus, thus causing a large excess of male offspring. Within a population meiotic drive selects for insensitive response alleles to which the anti-DENV effector gene would need to be linked. However, in many populations of *Ae. aegypti* the meiotic driver M^D seems to be absent and females of only relatively few natural populations appear to be sensitive to it. Consequently, this drive system is not universally applicable for *Ae. aegypti* in the field. Furthermore, its molecular biology in mosquitoes is unknown. The principle of underdominance implies that hybrids of two strains, the one of them more-fit than the other, would be less-fit than either one of them (*74, 75, 76*). Nevertheless, if the less-fit strain is far more abundant than the more-fit strain the former would eventually outcompete the latter. A transgene that reduces the fitness of offspring resulting from mating between wild types and released transgenic mosquitoes would be fixed in the population if the released transgenic parents would greatly outnumber the local wild types. Thus, to make use of an underdominance effect it would be necessary to mass release mosquitoes harboring the anti-DENV effector. The inheritance pattern of the gram-negative endosymbiont *Wolbachia* suggests it to be a potential genetic drive system (*77, 78*). *Wolbachia* is naturally infecting *Ae. albobictus* and *Ae. aegypti* mosquitoes have been artificially infected with it under laboratory conditions. *Wolbachia* can cause cytoplasmic incompatibility so that progeny of *Wolbachia* infected males and non-infected females would be non-viable. Since infected females breed normally with infected or non-infected males, *Wolbachia* establishes a reproductive advantage for the former, and this way acts as a gene drive mechanism. So far however, *Wolbachia* has not been successfully coupled with a transgene to be driven through a mosquito population, which is an important requisite to use this system for population replacement strategies in the field. Homing endonuclease genes (HEG) are selfish genes with unique properties and were discovered among fungi, bacteria and viruses (*79*, *80*). Homing endonucleases recognize and cleave 18-30 nt sequence motifs found on chromosomes that do not contain a copy of themselves. The homologous DNA repair machinery of the cell recognizes the double stranded break and repairs it by inserting a copy of the HEG in the center of its recognition sequence, this way destroying the recognition motif. HEG recognition sequences have been not found among the genome of *Ae. aegypti.* Thus, for use in mosquitoes a HEG needs to be modified to recognize a specific motif of interest conserved among the genomic DNA of various *Ae. aegypti* populations. If this could be achieved HEG would be a very powerful gene drive system leading to early-on fixation within a population. It could be also used for population reduction strategies via endogenous gene disruption. Medea is a selfish maternal effect lethal factor that has been discovered in *Tribolium* sp. (*81*). So far the molecular mechanism behind Medea in *Tribolium* is not well understood. Medea causes maternal-effect lethality to all progeny that do not inherit a copy of it, thus upon invading a population the factor will become fixed. Recently, a synthetic Medea system was successfully engineered for Drosophila (*82*) by silencing a maternally expressed gene that is essential for embryogenesis which is coupled to a rescuing gene expressed in the zygote. The essential gene, *Myd88*, is silenced in all oocytes produced by the female. Only those embryos that inherited a Medea bearing chromosome from the male, female or both parents are able to rescue the gene through the zygotically expressed antidote which consists of a copy of the *Myd88* ORF. Currently, the same research group that engineered Medea for Drosophila is trying to adopt this system for *Ae. aegypti*.

Taken together, for the successful implementation of the population replacement strategy in the field the transgene containing an anti-DENV effector needs to be tightly linked to a gene drive system. So far, there is no such system readily available for *Ae. aegypti*. However, we believe that Medea could be a promising candidate for an *Ae. aegypti* specific gene drive system in the near future.

References

1. Monath, T. P. *Proc. Natl. Acad. Sci. USA* **1994**, *91*, 2395-2400.
2. Gubler, D. J. *Emerg. Infect. Dis*. **1998**, *4*, 442-450.
3. Calisher, C. H. *Emerg. Infect. Dis.* **2005**, *11*, 738-739.
4. World Health Organization. *Prevention and control of dengue and dengue hemorrhagic fever.* WHO regional publication, SEARO, Geneva, 1999; pp.
5. Clyde K.; Kyle, J. L.; Harris, E. *J. Virol.* **2006**, *80*, 11418-11431.
6. Hombach, J.; Cardosa, M. J.; Sabchareon, A.; Vaughn, D. W.; Barrett, A. D. *Vaccine* **2005**, 25, 4130-4139.
7. Gubler, D. J. *Clin. Microbiol. Rev*. **1998**, *11*, 480-496.
8. Rodriguez, M. M.; Bisset, J. A.; Fernandez, D. *J. Am. Mosq. Control Assoc.* **2007**, *23*, 420-429.
9. Da-Cunha, M. P.; Lima, J. B.; Brogdon, W. G.; Moya, G. E.; Valle, D. *Mem. Inst. Oswaldo Cruz* **2005**, *100,* 441-444.
10. Lindenbach, B. D.; Thiel, H.-J.; Rice, C. M. In *Fields Virology*; Knipe, D. M.; Howley, P. M., Eds.; Fifth Edition; Lippincott, Williams & Wilkins: Philadelphia, PA, 2007; Vol.1, pp 1101-1152.
11. Chambers, T. J.; Weir, R. C.; Grakoui, A.; McCourt, D. W.; Bazan, J. F.; Fletterick, R. J.; Rice, C. M. *Proc. Natl. Acad. Sci. USA* **1990**, *87,* 8898-8902.

12. Rice, C. M. *Adv. Exp. Med. Biol.* **1996**, *397*, 31-40.
13. Blair C. D.; Adelman, Z. N.; Olson, K. E. *Clin. Microbiol. Rev.* **2000**, *13*, 651-661.
14. Hardy, J. L. In *The Arboviruses;* Monath, T. P., Ed.; CRC Press, Boca Raton, FL, 1988; Vol. 1, pp. 87-126.
15. Linthicum, K. J.; Platt, K.; Myint, K. S.; Lerdthusnee, K.; Innis, B. L.; Vaughn, D. W. *Med. Vet. Entomol.* **1996**, *10*, 87-92.
16. Salazar, M. I.; Richardson, J. H.; Sanchez-Vargas, I.; Olson, K. E.; Beaty, B. J. *BMC Microbiol.* **2007**, *30*, 7:9.
17. Bennett, K. E.; Olson, K. E.; Munoz Mde, L.; Fernandez-Salas, I.; Farfan-Ale, J. A.; Higgs, S.; Black, W. C.; Beaty, B. J. *Am. J. Trop. Med. Hyg.* **2002**, *67*, 85-92.
18. Black W.; Bennett K.; Gorrochotegui-Escalante N.; Barillas-Mury C.; Fernandez-Salas I.; de Lourdes Munoz M.; Farfan-Ale J.; Olson K.; Beaty B. *Arch. Med. Res.* **2002**, *33*, 379-388.
19. Bosio, C. F.; Fulto, R. E.; Salasek, M. L.; Beaty, B. J.; Black, W. C. *Genetics* **2000**, *156*, 687-698.
20. Bennett, K. E.; Flick, D.; Fleming, K. H.; Beaty, B. J.; Black, W. C. *Genetics* **2005**, *170*, 185-194.
21. Myles, K. M.; Pierro, D. J.; Olson, K. E. *J. Med. Entomol.* **2004**, *41*, 95-106.
22. Campbell, C. L.; Keene, K. M.; Brackney, D. E.; Olson, K. E.; Blair, C. D.; Wilusz, J.; Foy, B. D. *BMC Microbiology* **2008** *8:47.*
23. Wang, X.-H.; Aliyari, R.; Li, W.-X.; Kim, K.; Carthew, R.; Atkinson, P.; Ding, S.-W. *Science* **2006**, *312*, 452-454.
24. Galiana-Arnoux, D.; Dostert, C.; Schneemann, A.; Hoffmann, J. A.; Imler, J. L. *Nat. Immunol.* **2006**, *7*, 590-597.
25. Van Rij, R. P.; Saleh, M. C.; Berry, B.; Foo, C.; Houk, A.; Antoniewski, C.; Andino, R. *Genes Dev.* **2007**, *20*, 2985-2995.
26. Lee, Y.-S.; Nakahara, K.; Pham, J.-W.; Kim, K.; He, Z.; Sontheimer, E. J.; Carthew, R. W. *Cell* **2004**, *117*, 69-81.
27. Liu, Q.; Rand, T. A.; Kalidas, S.; Du, F.; Kim, H. E.; Smith, D. P.; Wang, X. *Science* **2003** *301*, 1921-1925.
28. Liu, X.; Jiang, F.; Kalidas, S.; Smith, D.; Liu, Q. *RNA* 2006, *12*, 1514-1520.
29. Matranga, C.; Tomari, Y.; Shin, C.; Bartel, D.P.; Zamore, P. D. *Cell*, **2006**, *123*, 607-620.
30. Hammond, S. M.; Boettcher, S.; Caudy, A. A.; Kobayashi, R.; Hannon, G. J. *Science* **2001**, *293*, 1146-1150.
31. Keene, K. M.; Foy, B. D.; Sanchez-Vargas, I.; Beaty, B. J.; Blair, C. D.; Olson, K. E. *Proc. Natl. Acad. Sci. USA* **2004**, *101*, 17240-17245.
32. Franz, A. W. E.; Sanchez-Vargas, I.; Adelman, Z. N.; Blair, C. D.; Beaty, B. J.; James, A. A.; Olson, K. E. *Proc. Natl. Acad. Sci. USA* **2006**, *103*, 4198-4203.
33. Adelman, Z. N.; Anderson, M. A.; Morazzani E. M.; Myles, K. M. *Insect Biochem. Mol. Biol.* **2008**, *38*, 705-713.
34. Sanchez-Vargas, I.; Scott, J. C.; Poole, B. K.; Franz, A. W. E.; Barbosa Solomieu, V.; Wilusz, J.; Olson, K. E.; Blair, C. D. *PLoS Pathog.* **2008**, *in press.*

35. Sanchez-Vargas, I.; Travanty, E. A.; Keene, K. M.; Franz, A. W. E.; Beaty, B. J.; Blair, C. D.; Olson, K. E. *Virus Res.* **2004**, *102*, 65-74.
36. Xi, Z.; Raminez, J. L.; Dimopoulos, G. *PLoS Pathog.* **2008**, *4*, e1000098
37. Adelman, Z. N.; Blair, C. D.; Carlson, J. O.; Beaty, B. J.; Olson, K. E. *Insect Mol. Biol.* **2001**, *10*, 265-273.
38. Adelman, Z. N.; Sanchez-Vargas, I.; Travanty, E. A.; Carlson, J. O.; Beaty, B. J.; Blair, C. D.; Olson, K. E. *J. Virol.* **2002**, *76*, 12925-12933.
39. Morris A. C.; Eggleston, P.; Crampton, J. M. *Med. Vet. Entomol.* **1998**, *3*, 1-7.
40. Grossman, G. L.; Rafferty, C. S.; Clayton, J. R.; Stevens, T. K.; Mukabayire, O.; Benedict, M. Q. *Insect Mol. Biol.* **2001**, *10*, 597-604.
41. Perera, O. P.; Harrell II, R. A.; Handler, A. M. *Insect Mol. Biol.* **2002**, *11*, 291-297.
42. Catteruccia, F.; Nolan, T.; Loukeris, T. G.; Blass, C.; Savakis, C.; Kafatos, F. C.; Crisanti, A. *Nature* **2000**, *405*, 959-962.
43. Jasinskiene, N.; Coates, C. J.; Benedict, M. Q.; Cornel, A. J.; Rafferty, C. S.; James, A. A. *Proc. Natl. Acad. Sci. USA* **1998**, *95*, 3743-3747.
44. Allen, M. L.; O'Brochta, D. A.; Atkinson, P. W.; Levesque, C. S. *J. Med. Entomol.* **2001**, *38*, 701-710.
45. Fraser M. J.; Ciszczon, T.; Elick, T.; and Bauser, C. *Insect Mol. Biol.* **1996**, *5*, 141-151.
46. Loukeris, T. G.; Arca, B.; Livadaras, I.; Dialektaki, G.; Savakis, C. *Proc. Natl. Acad. Sci. U S A.* **1995**, *92*, 9485-9489.
47. Hartl., D. L.; Lohe, A. R.; Lozovskaya, E. R. *Ann. Rev. Genetic.* **1997**, *31*, 337-358.
48. O'Brochta, D. A.; Sethuraman, N.; Wilson, R.; Hice, R. H.; Pinkerton, A. C.; Levesque, C. S.; Bideshi, D. K.; Jasinskiene, N.; Coates, C. J.; James, A. A.; Lehane, M. J.; Atkinson, P. W. *J. Exp. Biol.* **2003**, *206*, 3823-3834.
49. Horn C.; Wimmer, E. A. *Dev. Genes. Evol.* **2000**, *210*, 630-637.
50. Wendell M. D.; Wilson, T. G.; Higgs, S.; Black, W. C. *Insect Mol. Biol.* **2000**, *9*, 119-125.
51. Thomas, D. D.; Donnelly, C. A.; Wood, R. J.; Alphey, L. A. *Science* **2000**, *287*, 2474-2476.
52. Alphey, L. *Insect Biochem. Mol. Biol.* **2002**, *32*, 1243-1247
53. Phuc, H. K.; Andreasen, M. H.; Burton, R. S.; Vass, C.; Epton, M. J.; Pape, G.; Fu, G.; Condon, K. C.; Scaife, S.; Donnelly, C. A.; Coleman, P. G.; White-Cooper, H.; Alphey, L. *BMC Biology* **2007**, 5:11.
54. Handler, A. M.; Harrell, R. A. *Biotechniques* **2001**, *31*, 824-828.
55. Travanty, E. A.; Adelman, Z. N.; Franz, A. W. E.; Keene, K. M.; Beaty, B. J.; Blair, C. D.; James, A. A.; Olson, K. E. *Insect. Biochem. Mol. Biol.* **2004**, *34,* 607-613.
56. Kokoza, V.; Ahmed, A.; Cho, W. L.; Jasinskiene, N.; James, A. A.; Raikhel, A. S. *Proc. Natl. Acad. Sci. USA* **2000**, *97*, 9144-9149.
57. Kokoza, V. A.; Martin, D.; Mienaltowski, M. J.; Ahmed, A.; Morton, C. M.; Raikhel, A. S. *Gene* **2001**, *274*, 47-65.
58. James, A. A.; Blackmer, K.; Marinotti, O.; Ghosn, C. R.; Racioppi, J. V. *Mol. Biochem. Parasitol.* **1991**, *44*, 245-253.

59. Coates, C. J.; Jasinskiene, N.; Pott, G. B.; James, A. A. *Gene* **1999**, *226*, 317-325.
60. Edwards, M. J.; Moskalyk, L. A.; Donelly-Doman, M.; Vlaskova, M.; Noriega, F. G.; Walker, V. K.; Jacobs-Lorena, M. *Insect Mol. Biol.* **2000**, *9*, 33-38.
61. Moreira, L. A.; Edwards, M. J.; Adhami, F.; Jasisnkiene, N.; James, A. A.; Jacobs-Lorena, M. *Proc. Natl. Acad. Sci. USA* **2000**, *97*, 10895-10898.
62. Pham, D. Q.-D.; Shaffer, J. J.; Chavez, C. A.; Douglass, P. L. *Insect Biochem. Mol. Biol.* **2003**, *33*, 51-62.
63. Adelman, Z. N.; Jasinskiene, N.; Vally, K. M.; Peek, C.; Travanty, E. A.; Olson, K. E.; Brown, S. E.; Stephens, J. L.; Knudson, D. L.; Coates, C. J.; James, A. A. *Transgenic. Research* **2004**, *13*, 411-425.
64. Niu, L.-L.; Kiley, L. M.; Dasgupta, R.; Kohler, P.; Christensen, B. M. *Insect Mol. Bol.* **2003**, *12*, 571-579.
65. Beerntsen, B. T.; Champagne, D. E.; Coleman, J. L.; Campos, Y. A.; James, A. A. *Insect Mol. Biol.* **1999**, *8*, 459-467.
66. Helliwell, C. A.; Waterhouse, P. M. *Methods Enzymol.* **2005**, *392*, 24-35.
67. Smith, N. A.; Singh, S. P.; Wang, M. B.; Stoutjesdijk, P. A.; Green, A. G.; Waterhouse, P. M. *Nature* **2000**, *407*, 319–320.
68. James, A. A. *Trends Parasitology* **2005**, *21*, 64-67.
69. Ribeiro; J. M.; Kidwell, M. G. *J. Med. Entomol.* **1995**, *31*, 10-16.
70. Carareto, C. M.; Kim, W.; Wojciechowski, M. F.; O'Grady, P.; Prokchorova, A. V.; Silva, J. C.; Kidwell, M. G. *Genetica* **1997**, *101*, 13-33.
71. Sweeny, T. L.; Barr, A. R. *Genetics* 1977, *88*, 427-446.
72. Cha, S.-J.; Mori, A.; Chadee, D. D.; Severson, D. W. *Am. J. Trop. Med. Hyg.* **2006**, *74*, 62-68.
73. Cha, S.-J.; Chadee, D. D.; Severson, D. W. *Am. J. Trop. Med. Hyg.* **2006**, *75*, 70-77.
74. Davis, S.; Bax, N.; Grewe, P. *J. Theor. Biol.* **2001**, *212*, 83-98.
75. Magori, K.; Gould, F. *Genetics* **2006**, *172*, 2613-2620.
76. Gould, F.; Magori, K.; Huang, Y. *Am. Scientist* **2006**, *94*, 238-246.
77. Sinkins, S. P.; Godfray, H. C. J. *Proc. R. Soc. Lond.* **2004**, *271*, 1421-1426.
78. Xi, Z.; Khoo, C.; Dobson, S. L. *Science* **2005**, *310*, 326-328.
79. Burt, A. *Proc. R. Soc. Lond.* **2002**, *270*, 921-928.
80. Windbichler, N.; Papathanos, P. A.; Catteruccia, F.; Ranson, H.; Burt, A.; Crisanti, A. *Nucl. Acids, Res.* **2007**, *35*, 5922-5932.
81. Beeman, R. W.; Friesen, K. S.; Denell, R. E. *Science* **1992**, *256*, 89-92.
82. Chen, C. H.; Huang, H.; Ward, C. M.; Su, J. T.; Schaeffer, L. V.; Guo, M.; Hay, B. A. *Science* **2007**, *316*, 597-600.

Chapter 10

Pharmacological Mapping of the Acetylcholinesterase Catalytic Gorge in Mosquitoes with *Bis*(n)-Tacrines

Troy D. Anderson[1], Sally L. Paulson[1], Dawn M. Wong[2], Paul R. Carlier[2], and Jeffrey R. Bloomquist[1]

Departments of [1]Entomology and [2]Chemistry, Virginia Polytechnic Institute and State University, Blacksburg, Virginia, U.S.A. 24061

New insecticides are needed for control of mosquitoes, such as *Anopheles gambiae*, the major vector of malaria. Acetylcholinesterase is a proven insecticide target site, but conventional organophosphate and carbamate compounds are plagued by concerns about human toxicity and resistance. A pharmacological approach with novel, bivalent *bis*(n)-tacrines was used to map the catalytic gorge of this enzyme from human and several mosquito species (*Anopheles gambiae*, *Culex restuans*, *Aedes aegypti*, and *Aedes albopictus*). We screened bivalent *bis*(n)-tacrines having methylene linkers from 2-12 carbons in length, where proper spacing would allow for high potency binding via interaction with both the catalytic and peripheral sites on the enzyme. The tacrine monomer had fairly similar potency across species (somewhat less for *Culex restuans*), indicating a common mode of binding at the catalytic site. A greater maximal potency for a *bis*(n)-tacrine was observed against human AChE than any of the mosquitoes tested. With the exception of *Anopheles gambiae*, the mosquitoes showed a clear tether length dependence, with tether length most critical in *Aedes aegypti*. This finding has implications for identifying the targeted amino acid residues in or near the gorge. Despite the greater potency of *bis*(n)-tacrines against vertebrate than mosquito acetylcholinesterase, the information gleaned from this study should help inform the molecular design of selective anticholinesterase insecticides in other chemical series.

Introduction

Mosquito vectored diseases cause extensive mortality in humans (*1*). By far, the most important vector borne disease is malaria, which is estimated to cause over 1 million deaths a year, world-wide. Other important diseases spread by mosquitoes include: dengue, yellow fever, and encephalitis, and the total number of global deaths from these diseases is estimated to be about 50,000/yr (*1*).

Acetylcholinesterase (AChE) is a serine hydrolase that hydrolyzes the neurotransmitter acetylcholine (ACh) in the nervous system of both insects and humans, and is a proven target site for organophosphate and carbamate insecticides (*2*). However, the widespread resistance of numerous insect species to these insecticides, and poor selectivity towards humans, limits the utility of these compounds in pest control programs. The gene encoding AChE in the marine fish *Torpedo californica* is homologous to the *ace-1* gene found in several insect species (*2,3*). Sussman *et al.* (*4*) first revealed that the tertiary structure of *T. californica* AChE contains a deep and narrow active site gorge (Fig. 1) with important subsites for ACh binding/hydrolysis and thereby possible interaction with inhibitors. These subsites include the catalytic triad, choline-binding site, peripheral anionic site, and the acyl-binding pocket (*5*), all of which appear to be conserved across many invertebrate species (*6*).

Inhibitors of AChE may interact with more than one site on the enzyme. For example, tacrine prevents the hydrolysis of ACh by occupying the active site near the catalytic serine (*7,8*). Similarly, inhibitors can impede cholinergic substrate access by binding to the peripheral site of AChE (*7,8*), located at the entrance of the catalytic gorge (Fig. 1). Inhibitors that simultaneously bind to the active and peripheral sites of AChE can occupy much of the gorge, and inhibit enzyme activity with high affinity (*7,8*). For example, bifunctional tacrine molecules (Fig. 2), optimally tethered with an alkylene chain, can interact simultaneously with both sites of the enzyme, resulting in greater potency compared to that of tacrine itself (*7*). Determining the optimal spacing of bivalent inhibitors by altering the tether length can act as a molecular ruler, and indicates the distance between the catalytic and peripheral sites, as shown previously for compounds anchored at the catalytic site (*9*).

We used pharmacological studies to explore the geometry of the active site gorge of AChE in several mosquito species. Specifically, the gorge was probed with a series of *bis*(n)-tacrines to provide some insights on gorge volume and the distance between the catalytic and peripheral sites. Results were compared to human AChE. The resulting information should be useful in the design of bivalent inhibitors of high potency and selectivity.

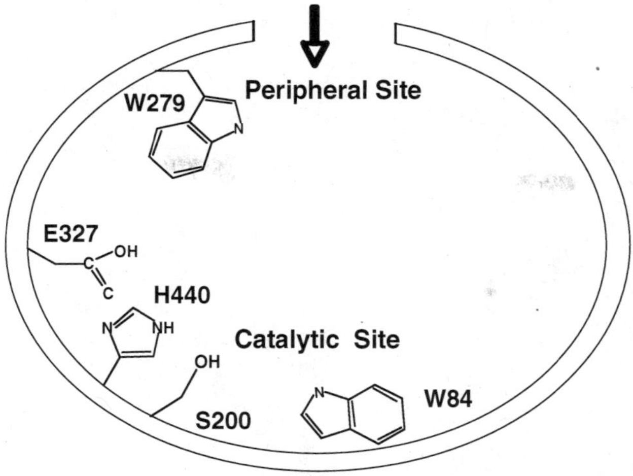

Figure 1. A simplified schematic representation of the AChE gorge with some key amino acids that define the peripheral aryl site and the catalytic active site. ACh enters the gorge at the peripheral site (arrow), and the hydrolysis products (acetate and choline) exit from the catalytic site.

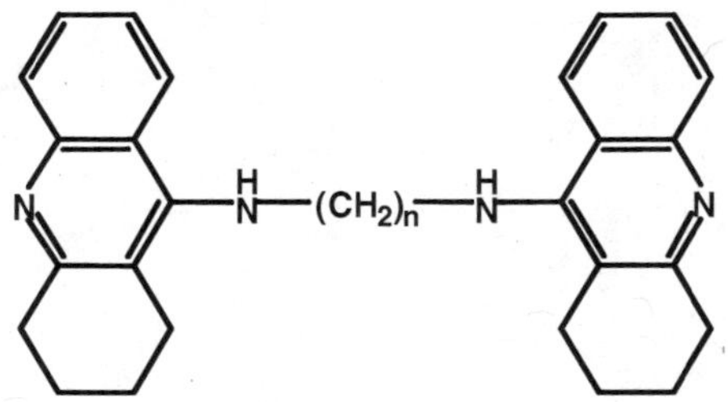

Figure 2. Chemical structure of the bis*(n)-tacrines used in this study, with 'n' representing the number of carbons that form the tether linkage. The* bis*(n)-tacrines were synthesized and purified to >99.5% using established methods (*10*).*

AChE Assay

Residual AChE activity was determined according to the method of Ellman *et al.* (*11*), with slight modifications. Malarial mosquitoes, *Anopheles gambiae* (G3 strain), were taken from colonies cultured in the Department of Entomology at Virginia Polytechnic Institute and State University. The mosquitoes *Aedes aegypti*, *Aedes albopictus*, and *Culex resutans* were collected from local wild populations. Adult mosquitoes were homogenized in 1 ml ice-cold 0.1 M sodium phosphate (pH 7.8) containing 0.3% (v/v) Triton X-100. The homogenate was centrifuged at 10,000 *g* for 15 min at 4 °C, and the supernatant was used for assay. The AChE preparations were pre-incubated with tacrine or each methylene-linked tacrine dimer (1-10,000 nM) for 10 min at room temperature. The residual AChE activity of the supernatant was measured using an enzyme kinetic microplate reader (Dynex Technologies, Chantilly, VA, USA) at 405 nm immediately after the addition of 5'5-dithiobis-(2-nitrobenzoic acid) (DTNB) and acetylthiocholine (ATCh). The final concentrations of DTNB and ATCh were 0.3 and 0.4 mM, respectively. Recombinant human AChE (lyophilized powder; Sigma-Aldrich, St. Louis, MO), with a quoted specific activity of 2790 U/mg, was diluted to 600 U/mL with 0.1 M sodium phosphate (pH 7.8) containing 0.3% (v/v) Triton X-100, frozen, and stored at −80 °C. Immediately prior to assay, a frozen human AChE sample was thawed and diluted 1000-fold with the same buffer before use. Nonlinear regression analysis of the residual AChE activity was used to determine the negative logarithm of IC_{50} for each inhibitor using Prism software (GraphPad Software Inc., San Diego, CA, USA).

Inhibition of AChE Activity by *Bis*(N)-Tacrines

Figure 3 and Table 1 reveal both similarities and differences in the responses of mosquito and human AChEs to inhibition by *bis*(n)-tacrines. The monomeric tacrine was among the least active compounds in each species, and with the exception of *Cx. restuans*, the sensitivity to this compound across species was similar (Table 1). This finding suggests that the binding of tacrine within the active site is comparable, but there is some difference in or near the catalytic site of *Cx. restuans* AChE that lowers affinity. Patterns of inhibition are visually apparent in Figure 3. In all cases, the IC_{50} decreased with increasing tether length compared to the monomer, and then increased again as tether length approached 12 methylenes, the maximum tested. There was a relatively flat response in *An. gambiae*, whereas the other species showed a greater tether length dependence reflected by a maximal potency at 7-8 methylenes. There is also a more steep tether length dependence in *Ae. aegypti* compared to any other species, since potency declines over 14-fold with a single carbon change from optimal tether length ($n = 8$) in *Ae. aegypti*, while potency declines < 3-fold with a one carbon change from optimal tether length for the others (Table 1). This difference suggests more efficient dual site binding in *Ae. aegypti* that rivals that of human AChE. Finally, the *bis*(n)-tacrines are uniformly more active against human AChE than any of the mosquito AChEs, at all tether lengths (Table 1). Thus, these compounds are negatively selective for mosquitoes. Other studies (*10, 12*) found that cockroach (*Blattella germanica*) and rat AChEs are, like *Ae. aegypti*, *Ae. albopictus* and *Cx. restuans*, most potently inhibited at a tether length of 7-8 carbons.

Although absent in human and minimal in *Ae. albopictus*, "bumps" were observed in the pattern of mosquito responses to the *bis*(n)-tacrines (Fig. 3). The most pronounced was at $n = 6$ in *An. gambiae*, with smaller ones at $n = 5$ in *Cx. restuans* and *Ae. aegypti*, suggesting a steric clash that impeded binding within the gorge. By way of comparison, the cockroach and rat enzymes have a "bump" at $n = 2$ tether length (*10, 12*), unlike any of the species studied here. This finding suggests that the gorge in these species is spatially constrained nearer the catalytic site.

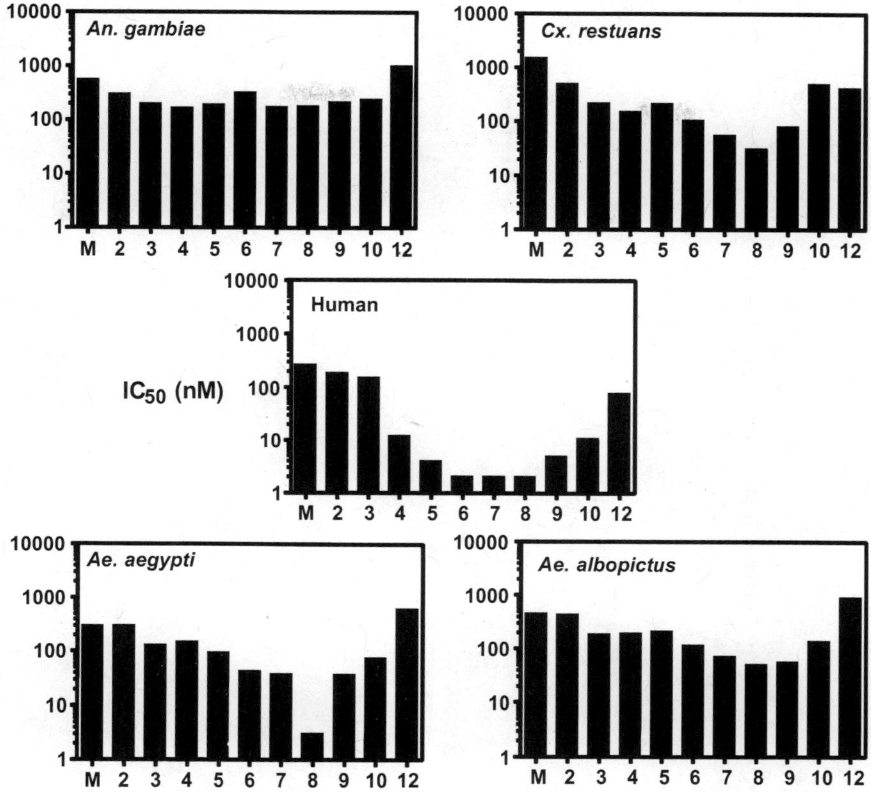

Figure 3. Comparison of IC_{50} values for tacrine monomer (M) and tether-length dependence of dimeric *bis*(n)tacrines, where numbers represent tether length in methylene units.

Table 1. Comparison of AChE inhibition for tacrine and *bis*(n)-tacrines on human, *Anopheles gambiae, Aedes aegypti, Aedes albopictus*, and *Culex restuans* AChE.

Compound	*Human* [a]*IC_{50} (nM)*	*An. gambiae* *IC_{50} (nM)*	*Ae. aegypti* *IC_{50} (nM)*	*Ae. albopictus* *IC_{50} (nM)*	*Cx. restuans* *IC_{50} (nM)*
Tacrine[b]	259 (223-301)	551 (478-635)	289 (257-326)	440 (396-490)	1,490 (1,226-1,811)
2	181 (133-246)	296 (223-394)	297 (251-350)	426 (376-483)	497 (410-602)
3	147 (123-174)	195 (143-264)	126 (116-136)	182 (162-205)	213 (165-273)
4	12 (10-13)	163 (133-201)	145 (133-157)	190 (169-214)	148 (123-179)
5	3.9 (3.4-4.4)	186 (155-222)	92 (89-95)	206 (170-249)	209 (176-247)
6	2.1 (1.9-2.3)	315 (278-358)	42 (39-45)	116 (98-137)	103 (91-117)
7	1.6 (1.1-2.3)	170 (146-197)	37 (33-41)	71 (59-85)	55 (44-68)
8	2.2 (1.9-2.6)	176 (153-203)	2.5 (2.1-3.0)	50 (44-58)	31 (23-41)
9	5.3 (4.5-6.3)	208 (192-225)	36 (30-43)	56 (46-69)	79 (63-100)
10	11 (9-12)	236 (217-257)	74 (69-80)	138 (110-173)	495 (344-712)
12	77 (65-90)	1,004 (1,000-1,070)	607 (543-679)	903 (826-987)	416 (330-525)

[a]Data are presented as IC_{50} (nM), the concentration at which 50% of AChE was inhibited, and their 95% confidence intervals in paretheses.

[b]Numbers are *n* in the term *bis*(n)-tacrine and represent the number of methylene units in the linker that tethers the tacrine moieties.

Protein Modeling

X-ray crystallographic studies of *bis*(7)-tacrine complexed with *Tc*AChE (PDB ID 2ckm), *(13)* found that one tacrine unit binds to the W84 choline-binding site (Fig. 4), sandwiched between the aromatic side chains of W84 and F330, at the bottom of the active-site gorge (*13).* This arrangement has also been observed in structures of monomeric tacrine (PDB ID 1ACJ) (*14*) and other tacrine-based bivalent inhibitors bound to *Tc*AChE (PDB ID 1ODC, 1UT6, 1Q83, 1Q84, 1ZGB. 1ZGC. 2CEK) (*13, 15-17*). We conclude that a similar binding mechanism operates in mosquitoes. The X-ray crystal structure of *bis*(7)-tacrine complexed to *Tc*AChE also reveals a π-complex sandwich of tacrine with W279 and Y70 at the peripheral site *(13*). Comparison of the *Tc*AChE and human AChE sequences suggests an identical binding mode would be realized for hAChE. The general lower overall potency of *bis*(n)-tacrines against mosquito AChEs relative to vertebrates may be due, in part, to the presence of I70 instead of the Y72 found in the human peripheral site (Fig. 4). We have proposed that such a substitution would diminish π-π/cation-π interaction at the peripheral site of *An. gambiae* AChE with the second tacrine moiety (*3*). However, such an explanation does not explain the high potency of *bis*(8)-tacrine against *Ae. aegypti*, which posses the same I70 substitution as *An. gambiae.* We are currently investigating enzyme-ligand interactions that could account for the high potency binding of this molecule in *Ae. aegypti*.

Conclusions

Mosquito species differ considerably in their responses to *bis*(n)-tacrines. Although these compounds are useful probes of the geometry of the AChE catalytic gorge, we do not view them as lead compounds, since they have no contact activity against insects (data not shown). The lack of toxicity is likely due to the presence of basic nitrogens that prevent penetration to the target site. Our studies found a greater overall potency for these compounds against human AChE than any of the mosquitoes tested, similar to a previous study comparing rat and German cockroach. The greater potency against vertebrate than insect AChE suggests structural and/or functional differences that creates possibilities for further structure-activity investigation. This speculation could be further investigated by using *Ala*-scanning site directed mutagenesis of residues thought to interact with tacrines, coupled with extensive *in silico* molecular modeling. Such studies could help inform the molecular design of selective anticholinesterase insecticides.

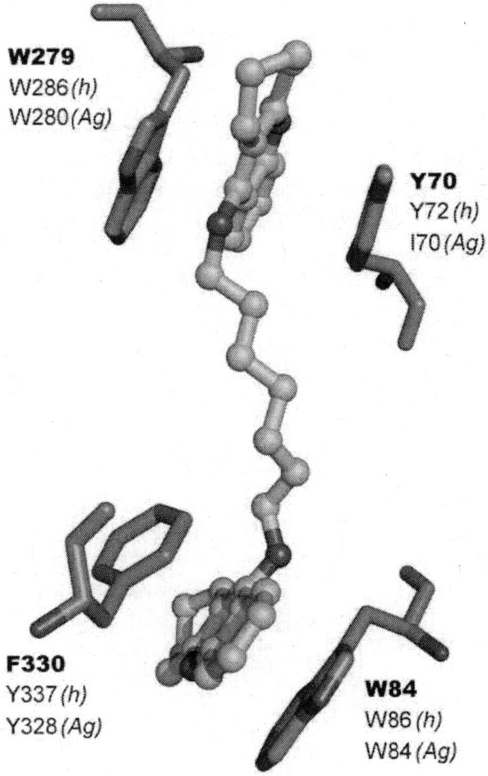

Figure 4. Molecular model using Pymol® of bis*(7)-tacine complexed with* Tc*AChE (bold text labels), including relevant amino acid residues of human and An. gambiae AChE. Figure is slightly modified from Carlier et al. (*3*).*

References

1. Hill, C. A.; Kafatos, F. C.; Stansfield, S. K.; Collins, F. H. *Nature Rev. Microbiol.* **2005**, *3*, pp 262-268.
2. Mutero, A.; Pralavoro, M.; Bride, J.-M.; Fournier, D. *Proc. Natl. Acad. Sci. USA* **1994**, *91*, pp. 5922-5926
3. Carlier, P.; Anderson, T.; Wong, D.; Hsu, D.; Hartsel, J.; Ma, M.; Wong, E.; Choudhury, R.; Lam, P.; Totrov, M.; Bloomquist, J. *Chemico-Biological Interactions* **2008**, *175* 368-375.
4. Sussman, J. L; Harel, M; Frolow, F; Oefner, C; Goldman, A; Toker, L; Silman, I. *Science* **1991**, *253*, pp 872-879.
5. Axelsen, P. H; Harel, M; Silman, I; Sussman, J. L. *Protein Sci.* **1994**, *3*, pp188-197.
6. Rowland, M; Tsigelny, I; Wolfe, M; Pezzementi, L. *Chemico-Biolog. Inter.* **2008**, Epub, in press.
7. Du, D. M; Carlier, P. R. *Curr. Pharm. Des.* **2004**, *10*, pp 3141-3156.
8. Lewis, W.; Green, L.; Grynszpan, F.; Radic, Z,; Carlier, P. R.; Taylor, P.; Finn, M. G.; Sharpless, K. B. *Angew. Chem. Int. Ed.* **2002**, *41*, pp 1053-1057.
9. Johnson, J.; Cusack, B.; Hughes, T.; McCullough, E.; Fauq, A.; Romanovskis, P.; Spatola, A.; Rosenberry, T.L. *J. Biol. Chem.* **2003**, *278*, pp 38948-38955.
10. Carlier, P. R; Han,Y. F; Chow, E. S-H; Li, C. P-L; Wang, H; Lieu, T. X; Wong, H. S; Pang, Y-P. *Bioorg. Med. Chem.* **1999**, *7*, pp 351-357.
11. Ellman G. L; Courtney, K. D; Andres, V; Featherstone, R. M. *Biochem. Pharmacol.* **1961**, *7*, pp 88-95.
12. Mutunga, J.; Anderson, T.; Wong , D.; Carlier, P.; Bloomquist, J. *ACS Symp. Ser.* **2008**, in press.
13. Rydberg, E. H; Brumshtein, B; Greenblatt, H. M; Wong, D. M; Shaya, D; Williams, L. D; Carlier, P. R; Pang, Y-P; Silman, I; Sussman, J. L. *J. Med. Chem.* **2006**, *49*, pp 5491-5500
14. Harel, M; Schalk, I; Ehret-Sabatier, L; Bouet, F; Goeldner, M; Hirth, C; Axelsen, P. H; Silman, I; Sussman, J. L. *Proc. Natl. Acad. Sci. USA.* **1993**, *90*, pp 9031-9035.
15. Bourne, Y.; Kolb, H. C.; Radic, Z.; Sharpless, K. B.; Taylor, P.; Marchot, P. *Proc. Natl. Acad. Sci. USA* **2004,** *101*, 1449-1454
16. Haviv, H.; Wong, D. M.; Greenblatt, H. M.; Carlier, P. R.; Pang, Y.-P.; Silman, I. *J. Am. Chem. Soc.* **2005,** *127*, 11029-11036.
17. Colletier, J. P; Sanson, B; Nachon, F; Gabellieri, E; Fattorusso, C; Campiani, G; Weik, M. *J. Am. Chem. Soc.* **2006**, *128*, pp 4526-4527.

Chapter 11

Olyset® net: a Long lasting Insecticidal Net for Vector Control

Takaaki Itoh[1], Yoshinori Shono[1], John R. Lucas[2] and Takao Ishiwatari[3]

1 Environmental Health Division, Sumitomo Chemical Co., Ltd., Tokyo, Japan
2 Sumitomo Chemical (U.K.) Plc, London, United Kingdom
3 Agricultural Chemicals Research Laboratory, Sumitomo Chemical Co., Ltd., Hyogo, Japan

Olyset® net is a long lasting insecticide treated mosquito net (LLIN) manufactured by Sumitomo Chemical Co., Ltd. The net material is polyethylene monofilament fibre, incorporated with permethrin 2% (w/w). Short exposure to Olyset® netting results in bite inhibition activity and rapid knockdown of mosquitoes. Field evaluations have shown that Olyset® net is an effective tool for controlling not only malaria but also dengue fever and leishmaniasis.

Introduction

Long –lasting insecticidal mosquito nets (LLINs) which retain activity for at least 3 years are recommended for malaria control by the World Health Organization (*1*).

Olyset® net is an LLIN manufactured by Sumitomo Chemical Co. Ltd. The net material is polyethylene monofilament fibre, incorporated with 2% w/w permethrin as the active ingredient (*2*). Olyset® net was the first LLIN to be submitted to the WHO Pesticides Evaluation Scheme (WHOPES) for evaluation, and the only LLIN currently fully recommended by WHO (*3*). In this paper we describe the biological efficacy and field evaluation of Olyset® net.

Contact Effect of Olyset® Net on Mosquitoes

We investigated the effects of short exposure to the net on the blood feeding behavior of mosquitoes. The method for testing is shown in Figuer 1. A piece of Olyset® net affixed to a plywood panel was placed in a mosquito cage, and a plastic dish with a 1 cm diameter hole in it was placed upside down on the Olyset® net. Five adult female yellow fever mosquitoes (*Aedes aegypti* (L.)) were confined inside the dish for three minutes during which time they came in contact with the net. Afterwards, the dish was removed, and the mosquitoes were allowed to fly freely inside the cage. After one minute, a hand was inserted into the cage, and the number of mosquitoes landing on the hand to feed was counted for one minute (when mosquitoes landed on the hand, the hand was shaken to prevent actual biting).

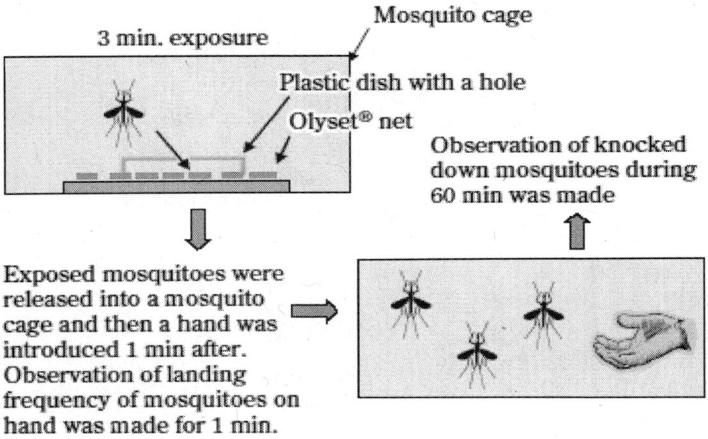

Figure 1. Short exposure test method to determine the effect of Olyset® net on the biting behavior of female Aedes aegypti.

The number of knocked down mosquitoes in the cage was also observed for 60 minutes. The number of landings on the hand and the knockdown results are shown in Figures 2 and 3 respectively. When the net was untreated, 40 insect landings per minute were observed, but with the Olyset® net, this fell to only five landings per minute. Knockdown results are recorded in Figure 2, which show significant levels of knockdown 10 minutes after contact, with some insects affected after 1 – 2 minutes. Observations indicated that mosquitoes that were in contact with Olyset® net for a short period of time were not able to recognize or respond to the host and did not show the probing activity normally associated with blood feeding insects .

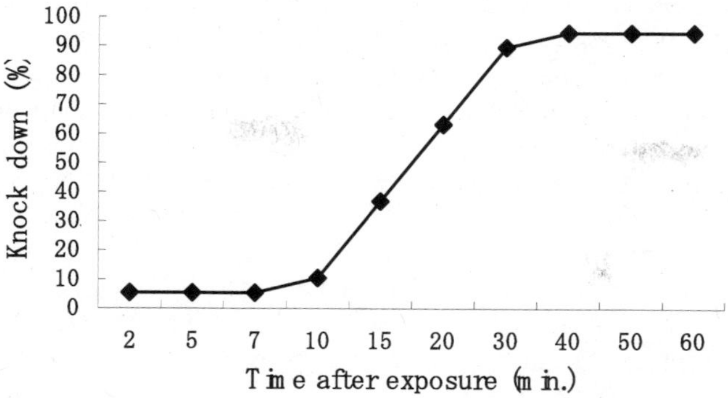

Figure 2. Knock down rate of Ae. aegypti after 3 minutes exposure to Olyset® net.

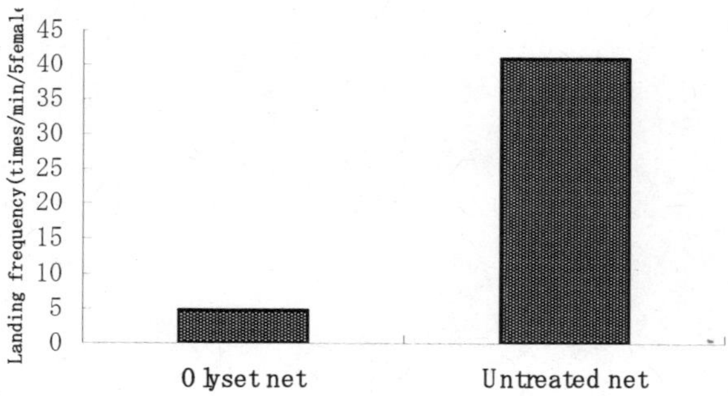

Figure 3. Landing frequency of Ae. aegypti after 3 minutes exposure to Olyset® net.

A Field Trial to Control Malaria in Cambodia

A field trial to control malaria was carried out by the National Malaria Center in a forested area 650 km northwest from Phnom Penh from June through December 1994 (*4*). The malaria vectors in this area are *Anopheles dirus* (Peyton and Harrison) and *Anopheles minimus* (Theobald). Malaria infections are approximately 60% falciparum malaria, 30% vivax malaria with about 10% mixed infections . There were 860 residents of the village where the Olyset® net was distributed and there were 1,000 residents in the village where untreated conventional mosquito nets were distributed. In an entomological survey conducted for two consecutive nights each month, mosquitoes were collected and their parous rate was determined. For an epidemiological survey, the changes in the positive rate for malaria were examined by blood tests in 50 pre-selected children under 5 years old and 50 children 5 years old or older once per month. Out of the large amount of data, the transitions in the parous rate for *Anopheles dirus* are shown in Figure 4. The parous rate means the ratio of mosquitoes in the mosquito population that have experienced oviposition. In other words, a high parous rate means a high proportion of older mosquitoes in the population. After the malaria parasites have been taken into the body of the mosquito through feeding on an infected person, they develop to the sporozoite stage during two weeks inside the body of the mosquito and reach the salivary glands of the mosquito; then the parasite can be transmitted to a healthy person by injecting the sporozoites at the time of blood feeding. Therefore, having a large number of older mosquitoes means that the risk of a malarial infection is high. From Figure 4, it can be confirmed that the parous rate for the villages where Olyset® nets were distributed quickly dropped in comparison with the changes in the parous rate in the villages where untreated mosquito nets were distributed. It was suggested that mosquitoes were killed in contact with Olyset® nets, and an increase in the proportion of younger mosquitoes present was exhibited. Expanding on this further, it shows that as the number of mosquitoes that had reached the sporozoite stage became lower, and the risk of infection was decreased. Figure 5 shows the results of blood inspection in children. In the villages where Olyset® net was distributed, the positive rate for malaria became zero after three months. The positive rate for the villages where the untreated mosquito nets were distributed did not go to zero. From these field trials, it is clear that it is possible to effectively reduce or prevent malaria transmission through the use of Olyset® nets.

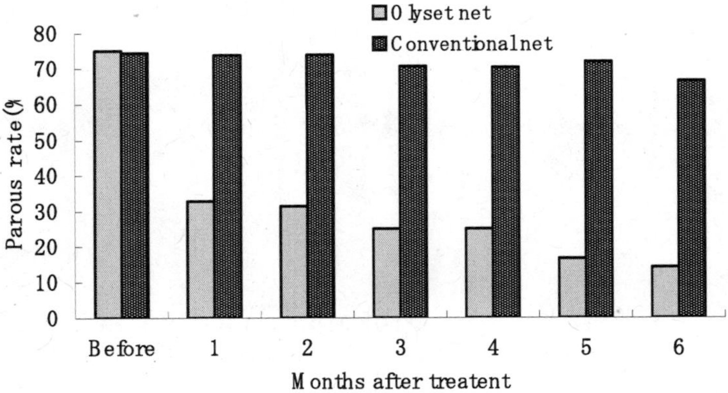

Figure 4. Changes in parous rate of Anopheles dirus collcted inside house after Olyset® net treatment. (Drawn by the data from reference 4).

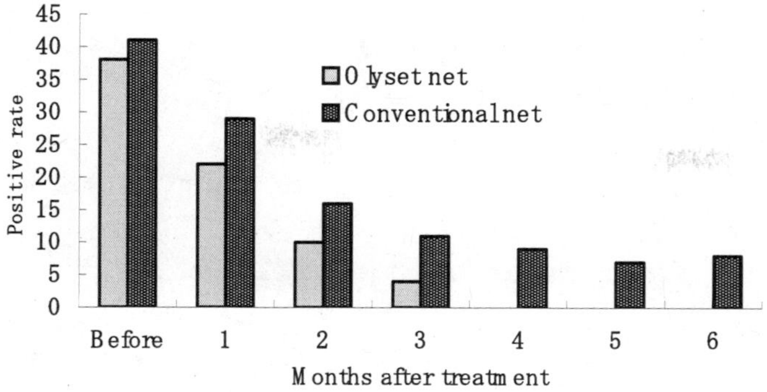

Figure 5. Changes in malaria positive rate in children after Olyset® net treatment **(Drawn by the data from reference 4).**

Several studies have been conducted to evaluate the longevity of Olyset® net in practical use conditions. Tami et al. collected 7 year old used Olyset® nets from two Tanzanian villages and examined insecticide dosage and biological efficacy. . The results show that permethrin content was 33-41% of the original content and these nets still exhibited a high knock down rate (*5*). Malima et al. examined insecticidal efficacy of seven-year old Olyset® nets in Tanzania and these used nets inhibited blood feeding by more than 95 % in tunnel tests (*6*). These results demonstrate that Olyset® nets still maintain insecticidal efficacy after 7 years under practical use conditions.

Olyset® Net for Dengue and Leishmaniasis Control

The effects of Olyset net on dengue and leishmaniasis have also been reported. Nugyen et al. carried out a field experiment for dengue vector control using Olyset® net screens. The screens were set to windows, door entrance and ventilation openings near the ceiling. After installing Olyset® screens, the density index of *Aedes aegypti* was reduced from 0.23 to zero in contrast to the control area where the index increased (Figure 6). The larval Breteau Index and larval house index was also reduced to undetectable levels in the experimental area (*7*).

Emani et al. used Olyset® net for leishmaniasis control in Iran. The results showed lower indoor density of *P. papatasi* Scopoli in the intervention area compared to the control area. From an epidemiological standpoint, there was a 97% reduction in anthroponotic cutaneous leishmaniasis (ACL) incidence compared to the control area (Figure 7) (*8*).

These results strongly indicate that Olyset® net would be an important tool for dengue and leishmaniasis control.

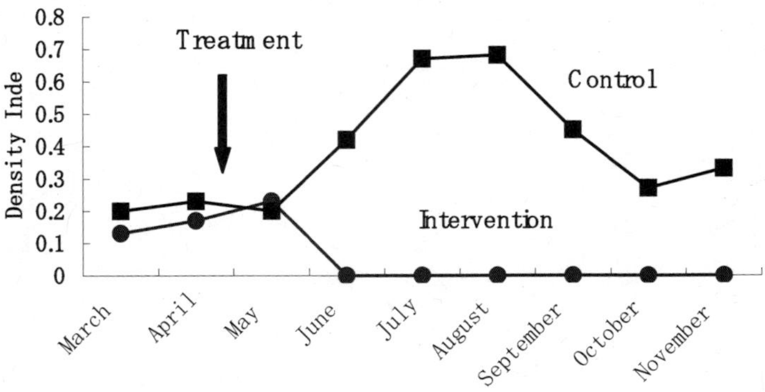

Fig. 6 Change in landing rate of Aedes aegypti in Olyset® net screen treated and untreated areas in Vietnam . (Drawn by the data from reference 7)

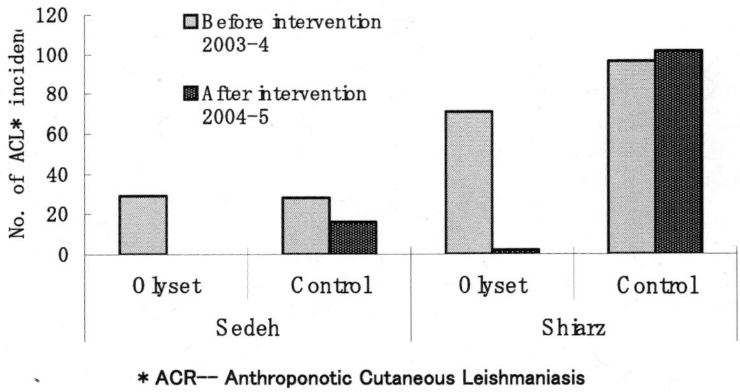

Figure 7. Epidemiological survey for field trial of Olyset® net to control leishmaniasis in Iran. (Drawn by the data from reference 8)

Conclusiton

Short exposure to Olyset® net results in significant bite inhibition activity and rapid knock down of mosquitoes. Field evaluations have shown that Olyset® net is an effective tool for controlling not only malaria but also dengue fever and leishmaniasis. As may be anticipated from these favorable results, Olyset® net is already being used in various situations for controlling vector borne diseases.

References

1. WHO. Global Malaria Program, WHO Position Statement 2007. Geneva, WHO. http://www.who.int/malaria/docs/itn/ITNspospaperfinal.pdf
2. Taklehaimanot A. ; Sachs J.D. ; Curtis C. ; *Lancet*, **2007**, *369:* 884
3. WHO/CDS/WHOPES/**2001**.4 16pp L
4. Cheang, Y. ; Sandy L. ; National Malaria Center, Phnom Penh, Cambodia, **1994**
5. Tami A. ; Mubyazi G. ; Talbert A. ; Mshinda H. ; Duchon S. ; Lengeler C. ; *Malararia Journal* **2004**, *3*, 19
6. Malima R.; Magesa S. ; Tunga P. ; Mwingira V. ; Magogo F. ; Sudi W. ; Mosha F. ; Curtis C. ; Maxwell C. ; Rowland M. ; *Malaria Journal* **2008**, *7*, 38
7. Nguyen H. T.; Tien T. V. ; Tien N. C. ; Ninh T. U. ; Hoa N. T.; *Dengue Bulletin* **1998** *20,* 87
8. Emami M. M. ; Yazdi M. ; Bashardoust N.; WHO Eestern Mediterrnean Region, Project No: SGS04-76, **2006**

Chapter 12

Biological Efficacy of Metofluthrin, a New Pyrethroid Insecticide, Highly Effective against Mosquitoes

Takao Ishiwatari[1], Masayo Sugano[1], John R. Lucas[2], and Yoshinori Shono[3]

[1] Agricultural Chemicals Research Laboratory, Sumitomo Chemical Co. Ltd., Hyogo, Japan.
[2] Sumitomo Chemical (U. K.) Plc, London, United Kingdom.
[3] Environmental Health Division, Sumitomo Chemical Co. Ltd., Tokyo, Japan.

Metofluthrin (commercial name: SumiOne®, Eminence®) is a novel pyrethroid insecticide developed by Sumitomo Chemical Co., Ltd. Metofluthrin has extremely high mosquito knockdown activity. In addition, metofluthrin has relatively high volatility and low mammalian toxicity. Thus, metofluthrin is applicable for use not only in existing mosquito control formulations such as coils and liquid vaporizers, but also in a variety of novel devices that do not require heating, such as fan vaporizers and paper and resin emanators. The present report describes the knockdown and bite inhibition activity of metofluthrin against mosquitoes in ambient temperature emanators in both laboratory and field trials

SumiOne® and Eminence® are registered trademarks of Sumitomo Chemical Company Limited.

Profile of Metofluthrin

Metofluthrin (SumiOne®, Eminence®) is a novel pyrethroid discovered by Sumitomo Chemical Co., Ltd. (*1*). The chemical name of metofluthrin is 2,3,5,6–tetrafluoro-4-methoxymethylbenzyl (*EZ*(*E*/*Z*=1/8))-(1*R*, 3*R*)-2,2-dimethyl-3-(prop-1-enyl)cyclopropanecarboxylate (Figure 1). Metofluthrin was registered in Japan in January 2005 and is currently under worldwide development for a variety of environmental health applications.

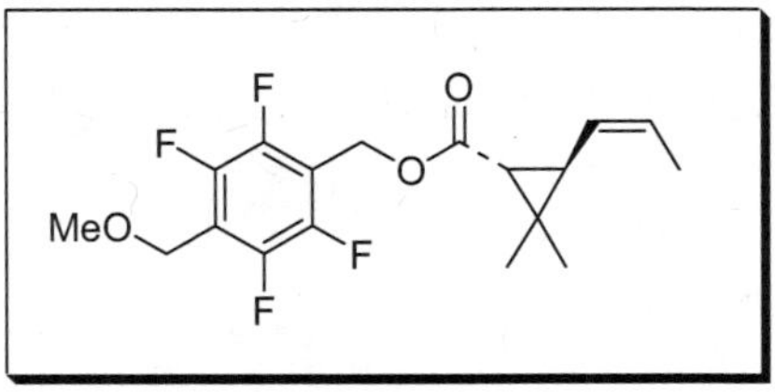

Figure 1. *Chemical Structure of Metofluthrin (SumiOne®, Eminence®)*

Metofluthrin has high lethal and knockdown activity against various pest insects especially mosquitoes. (*2*) Insecticidal efficacy of metofluthrin against four medically important mosquito species is between 19 and 49 times higher than that of *d*-allethrin by topical application method (Figure 2). Metofluthrin has a high volatility that is more than twice of *d*-allethrin (Table I) as well as low mammalian toxicity. Due to these characteristics metofluthrin is suitable for various formulations and devices, especially for use in the paper and resin devices that can emanate an active ingredient at ambient temperature without any energy source.

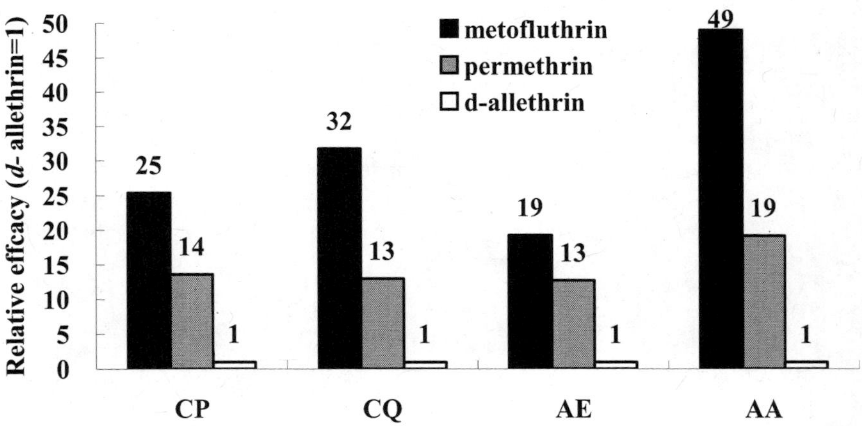

Figure 2. Insecticidal Efficacy against Mosquitoes, Topical Application Method CP: Culex pipiens pallens, CQ: Culex quinquefasciatus, AE: Aedes aegypti, AA: Aedes albopictus

Table I. Vapor Pressure of Insecticides

Insecticides	Vapor Pressure (Pa)*	Relative Vapor Pressure#
Metofluthrin	2.0×10^{-3}	2.5
d-allethrin	7.9×10^{-4}	1.0
Permethrin	7.3×10^{-6}	0.0093

* Gas chromatography method
# *d*-allethrin=1.0 (The larger the number the more volatile the compound)

Efficacy of Metofluthrin Ambient Temperature Emanators

Paper emanators

Typical ambient temperature emanators are containing active ingredient in a paper or resin substrate and the active ingredient is vaporized without heating or any other mechanical power. Insecticides used in such formulations must possess the following characteristics: vapour action at ambient temperature, high efficacy and a high level of safety to mammals. Metofluthrin meets all of these criteria.

In the first stage of development of the emanator, we evaluated efficacy of a device using paper as a substrate (Figure 3).

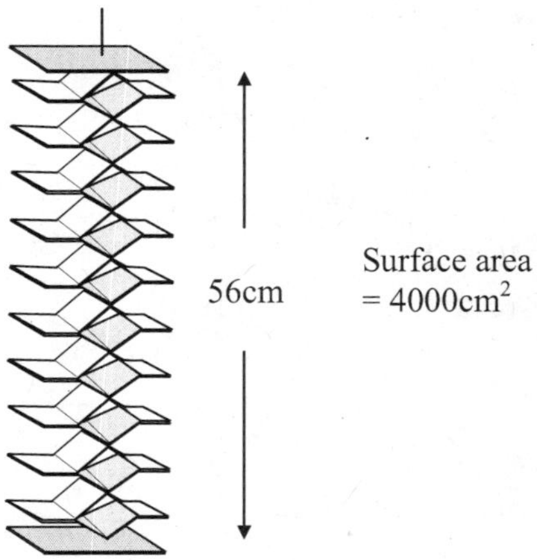

Figure 3. *Metofluthrin Paper Emanator*

Wind tunnel trial

To determine the efficacy of the paper emanator, we conducted laboratory tests in the USA using a wind tunnel and subsequently carried out field trials in Florida and Washington State (*3*). Paper emanator samples used in these tests contained 200mg of metofluthrin and were aged in a fume hood for 36 hours prior to test in order to confirm their duration of effectiveness. A wind tunnel was constructed of tubular steel covered with white translucent plastic (Figure 4). The wind tunnel was housed indoors (24-28 °C). A fan produced laminar airflow of approximately 0.18m/sec in the tunnel. A volunteer person and the paper emanator were positioned at given sites in the wind tunnel as shown in Figure 4. Emanator was hung in position E1 when tested singly and in position E1 and E2 when tested in pairs. Five minutes later, 40-50 *Aedes aegypti* (L.) blood-unfed adult females were released in the wind tunnel through an opening in the side of the tunnel (mosquito release point in Figure 4). Numbers of mosquitoes attracted to the volunteer were counted at 2 minute intervals up to 6 minutes. As shown in Table II, wind tunnel tests with aged emanators showed a marked reduction in both landing and biting activity.

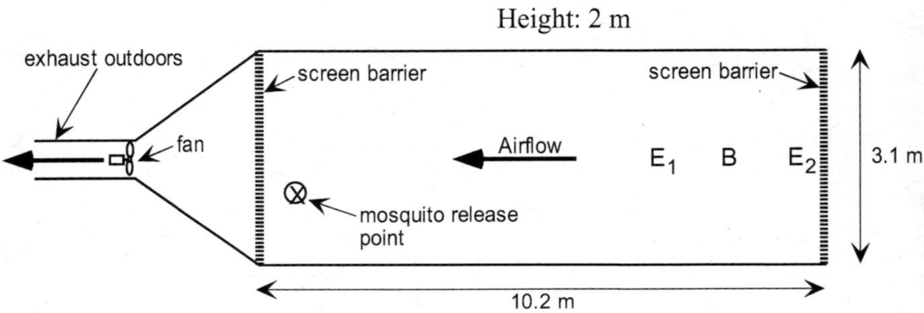

B = volunteer
E = emanators

Figure 4. *Top View of the Wind Tunnel (Reproduced from reference 3. Copyright 2007 The American Mosquito Control Association, Inc.)*

Table II. Efficacy of Metofluthrin Paper Emanators in the Wind Tunnel

Arrangement of Metofluthrin paper emanators	Total # of landings	% Reduction of landings	Total # of bites
One emanator, moving air	22	91.2	4
Two emanators, still air	24	90.4	1
No emanators, moving air	249	-	Too numerous to count

SOURCE: Reproduced from reference 3. Copyright 2007 The American Mosquito Control Association, Inc.

Field trials

Field trials were conducted in June and July 2004 in Washington State and Florida. Predominant species were *Aedes vexans* (Meigen) in Washington State and *Ochlerotatus taeniorhynchus* (Wiedemann) in Florida. Five volunteers were used per trial, wearing Tyvek® suits. Three replicate counts were made per volunteer. Use of skin applied repellents (e.g. DEET) etc. was prohibited. Mosquito landing rates were determined for a duration of 1 minute at intervals of 2 minutes up to 30 minutes. In Washington State there was almost no detectable air movement, with temperatures ranging between 16 and 27℃. In Florida wind speeds of up to 1.4mi/h and higher temperature were recorded (30-34℃). The test results demonstrate a dramatic decline in mosquito landing rates in both trials, as shown in Figure 5 and 6. These results demonstrate the excellent repellency of Metofluthrin paper emanators outdoors, even under heavy insect pressure.

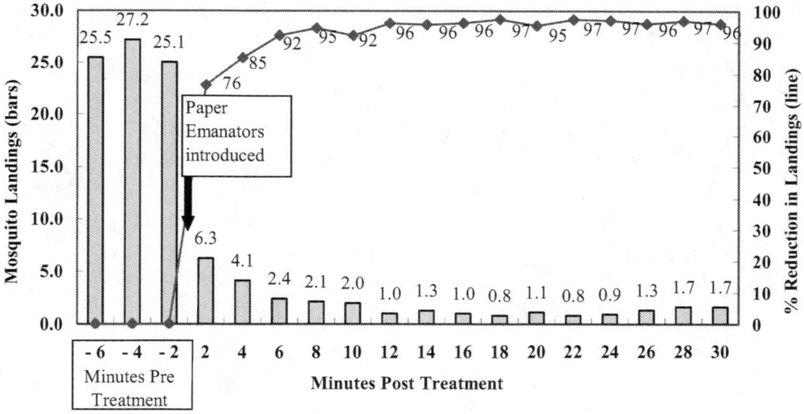

Figure 5. *Metofluthrin Paper Emanator Field Trials in Washington State (Reproduced from reference 3. Copyright 2007 The American Mosquito Control Association, Inc*

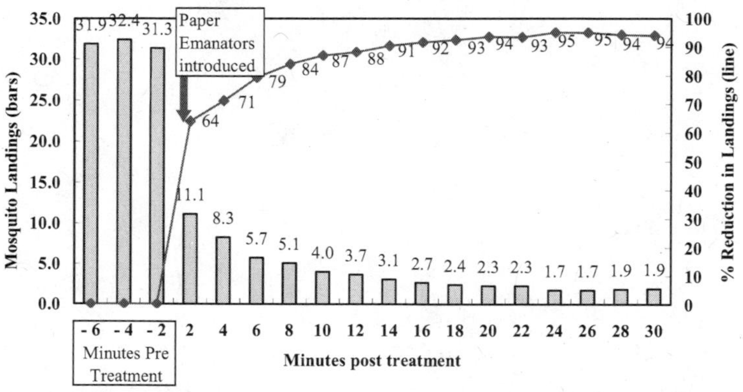

Figure 6. *Metofluthrin Paper Emanator Field Trials in Florida (Reproduced from reference 3. Copyright 2007 The American Mosquito Control Association, Inc.*

Practical tests using a similar paper emanators were conducted on Lombok Island in Indonesia and in Nagasaki, Japan. In a house on Lombok Island, a paper emanator impregnated with 200mg of metofluthrin exhibited repellent effects of 80% or greater against *Culex quinquefasciatus* Say and anopheline mosquitoes over a period of four weeks (*4*). In addition, in outdoor conditions on Lombok Island, these emanators exhibited superior repellent effects against *Cx. quinquefasciatus* as well as *Anopheles balabaciensis* Baisas and *An. sundaicus* (Rodenwaldt) (*5*). This emanator also exhibited high repellent activity against *Aedes albopictus* (Skuse) (*6*). From these results, we were able to confirm that metofluthrin paper emanators had excellent activity against various species of mosquitoes in practical conditions.

Resin emanator

After developing and evaluating paper emanator technology, we have continued to improve and develop new ambient temperature emanators by investigating alternative substrates on which metofluthrin is impregnated. Polyethylene resin is one of the most promising candidate materials for improving the performance and handling characteristics of ambient temperature emanators. This type of resin has some advantages compared with paper, such as improved and prolonged release characteristics, as well as being waterproof and far more durable than paper.

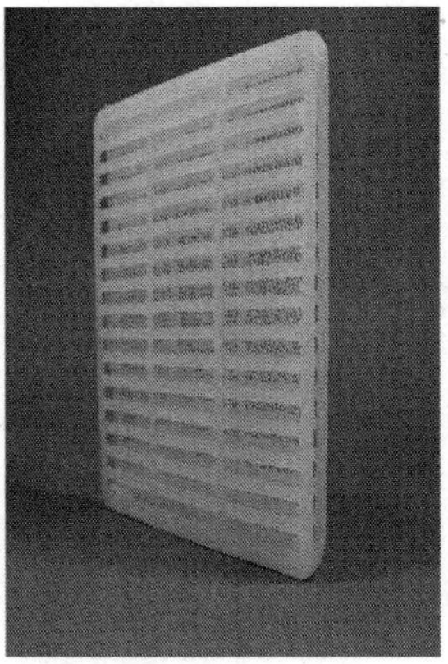

Figure 7. *Metofluthrin Resin Emanator*

To confirm the efficacy of metofluthrin resin emanators, we conducted a field trial in Japan. A polyethylene net incorporated with 185mg metofluthrin was folded and set in a plastic frame as shown in Figure 7. The plastic frame was used for making the emanator more compact and for protecting handlers from direct contact to the insecticide treated net. Field trials were conducted in Nagasaki, Japan. The predominant mosquito species was *Aedes albopictus*. The test method was almost the same as those of the trial conducted in the USA, as mentioned above. Under these test conditions metofluthrin resin emanators showed a dramatic decline in mosquito landing rates (Figure 8). These results demonstrate that the efficacy of resin emanators is similar to or better than that observed using paper emanators.

Practical tests using metofluthrin resin emanators with different shapes were subsequently conducted in Vietnam. Resin emanators containing 1g of metofluthrin exhibited excellent spatial repellent effects against both *Culex quinquefasciatus* and *Aedes aegypti* for at least six weeks (*7*).

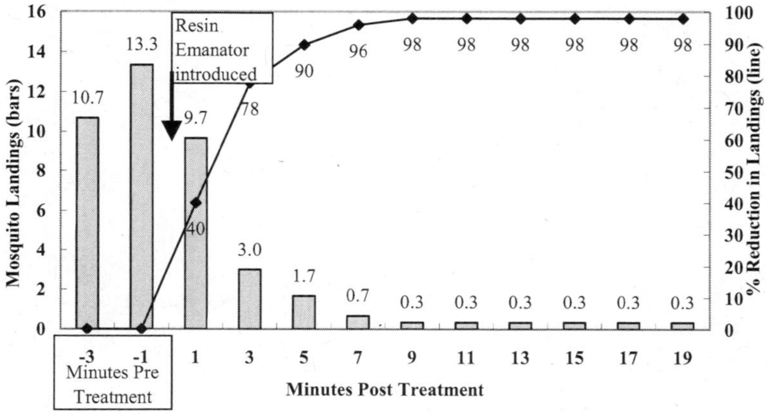

Figure 8. *Metofluthrin Resin Emanator Field Trials in Nagasaki, Japan*

Biting Inhibition Activity of Metofluthrin

The knockdown activity is usually evaluated in the laboratory as the criteria by which biological performance of mosquito control devices is compared. However, under more practical conditions, spatial repellency and biting inhibition activity are thought to more accurately reflect actual performance than knockdown activity. In order to evaluate biting inhibition activity in the laboratory we established a test method as follows: Two nylon mesh cages each containing a live chick were hung at 1.2 m above the floor in a test chamber ($28m^3$) and 100 adult blood-unfed female *Aedes aegypti* were released into the chamber (Figure 9). Five minutes after releasing mosquitoes, the number of insects attracted to each cage was counted. A mosquito coil was then ignited and set on a coil stand on the floor at a distance of 1.2 m from the two test cages. The number of mosquitoes attracted to the cages was then counted at designated intervals for the next 60 minutes. At the same time, the number of mosquitoes knocked down on the floor of the test chamber was also counted. This experiment was performed in accordance with the Guide for Animal Care and Use of Sumitomo Chemical Co. Ltd.

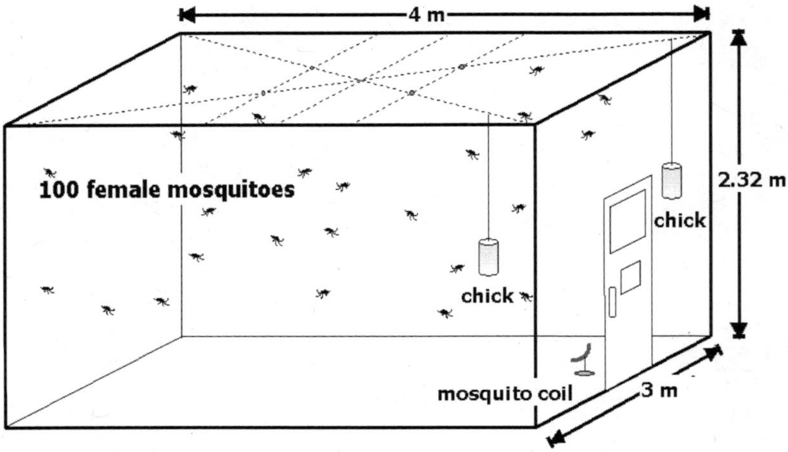

Figure 9. Test Method for Biting Inhibition against Aedes aegypti in Laboratory

Results are shown in Table III and IV. These results indicate that biting inhibition caused by metofluthrin occurred before insects were knocked down. Biting inhibition of metofluthrin was much more than 30 times higher than *d*-allethrin. This efficacy ratio is higher than that estimated when using knockdown as a performance criteria, which indicates that metofluthrin is approximately 30 times as active.

This data supports the excellent biting inhibition activity of metofluthrin noted in field trials.

Table III. Biting inhibition activity of Metofluthrin coil

Active ingredients	Conc. (%w/w)	Relative ratio	IT_{95} (min)
metofluthrin	0.01	1	7.2
d-allethrin	0.3	30	12.9

IT = Inhibition Time, IT_{95}(min): calculated time required for 95% biting inhibition (lower IT values mean higher efficacy)

Table IV. Knockdown activity of Metofluthrin coil

Active ingredients	Conc. (%w/w)	Relative ratio	KT_{50} (min)
metofluthrin	0.01	1	16.4
d-allethrin	0.3	30	15.9

KT = Knockdown Time, KT_{50}(min): calculated time required for 50% knockdown (lower KT values mean higher efficacy)

Summary

Metofluthrin is a newly developed highly effective vapor active pyrethroid having excellent insecticidal activity against mosquitoes. Due to these characteristics, metofluthrin is suitable for use in ambient temperature emanators that can be made from substrates as diverse as paper and plastic resin. Excellent biting inhibition activity of metofluthrin formulated into paper and resin emanators was demonstrated in both laboratory and field tests. This exciting new chemistry opens up new possibilities for the effective control of both nuisance biting insects as well as disease vectors.

References

1. K. Ujihara, T. Mori, T. Iwasaki, M. Sugano, Y. Shono, N. Matsuo, Biosci. Biotechnol. Biochem., 2004, 68, 170.
2. N. Matsuo, K. Ujihara, Y. Shono, T. Iwasaki, M. Sugano, T. Yoshiyama, S. Uwagawa, Sumitomo Kagaku, vol. 2005-II
3. J. R. Lucas, Y. Shono, T. Iwasaki, T. Ishiwatari. N. Spero, G. Benzon, J. Am. Mosq. Control Assoc., 2007, 23(1), 47.
4. H. Kawada, Y. Maekawa, Y. Tsuda, M. Takagi, J. Am. Mosq. Control Assoc., 2004, 20(3), 292.
5. H. Kawada, Y. Maekawa, Y. Tsuda, M. Takagi, J. Am. Mosq. Control Assoc., 2004, 20(4), 434.
6. T. Argutea, H. Kawada,, M. Takagi, Med. Entomol. Zool., 2004, 55(3): 211 – 216
7. H. Kawada, N. Yen., N. Hoa, T. Sang, N.Dan, M. Takagi, Am. J. Med. Hyg., 2005, 73(2), 350.

Chapter 13

An Inconvenient Truth of Pyrethroid - Does it have a promising future? -

Hitoshi Kawada

Institute of Tropical Medicine, Nagasaki University, Nagasaki, Japan

Pyrethroid is the general term for a group of chemicals that includes natural pyrethrins derived from Chrysanthemum flowers and their structurally related synthetic chemicals. Most of pyrethroids are highly nontoxic to mammals and possess high knockdown activity. Pyrethroid resistance is envisioned to be a major problem for the vector control program since, at present, there are no suitable chemicals substitutes for pyrethroids. Cross-resistance to knockdown agents, which are mainly used in mosquito coils and related products as spatial repellents, is the most serious concern. Since this is a global phenomenon, we have started to monitor the distribution of mosquito resistance to pyrethroids. The first pilot study was carried out in Vietnam. We periodically drove along the national road from the north end to the Mekong Delta in Vietnam and collected mosquito larvae from used tires. Simplified susceptibility tests were performed using the fourth instar larvae of *Aedes aegypti* (L.), *Aedes albopictus* (Skuse), and *Culex quinqufasciatus* (Say). The susceptibility of the abovementioned species against *d*-allethrin was lower in the southern part as compared to in northern part of Vietnam. Compared with the other species, *Ae. aegypti* demonstrated the most prominent reduction in susceptibility. For *Ae. aegypti*, significant increases in the susceptibility indices with decrease in the latitude of collection points were observed, indicating that the susceptibility of *Ae. aegypti* against *d*-allethrin was lower in the southern part including mountainous areas as compared to in the northern part of Vietnam. The significant correlation was observed between the susceptibility indices and the annual pyrethroid use for malaria control in *Ae. aegypti*. This might explain that the use of DDT and pyrethroids as residual treatment inside houses and pyrethroid-impregnated bed nets for malaria control are attributable to low pyrethroid susceptibility in *Ae. aegypti*. Such insecticide treatment appeared to have been intensively administered in the interior and along the periphery of human habitation areas where incidentally, the breeding and resting sites of *Ae. aegypti* are located. This might account for the strong selection pressure toward *Ae. aegypti* and not *Ae. albopictus*.

Pyrethroids and Mosquito Control

Development of insecticides

Insect pests are creatures that have emerged due to the activities of human beings and are harmful or disadvantageous from the human point of view. Sanitary pests and vectors of infectious diseases emerged as humans adopted communal living. Agricultural pests appeared as humans started to cultivate fields and grow crops. Food, clothing, and timber pests became apparent as humans started to store foods and clothes and to seek shelter. Nowadays, many creatures such as spiders, centipedes, millipedes, and ants have come to be hated and are categorized as nuisance pests because of the superfluous improvements in human lifestyle. In order to ensure human comfort or to improve it under more ideal conditions, humans have invented insecticides. Insecticides are, therefore, pest-regulating substances that have been invented by human beings for their own needs. What are the conditions or characteristics essential for a good insecticide? First of all, there will be no opposition that good insecticides should be as effective as possible. However, on the other hand, the development and manufacturing costs should be as low as possible. All too often, highly effective insecticides are also highly toxic to human beings or other organisms. Minimum toxicity, i.e., toxicity that is as low as possible is desirable. Moreover, insecticides should exert low environmental pressure, that is, have low environmental persistence and few adverse effects on the environment. Minimal effects on non-target organisms, including fish, insects, algae, and other creatures are also desirable. All the abovementioned characteristics should be considered while developing a new insecticide (Figure 1).

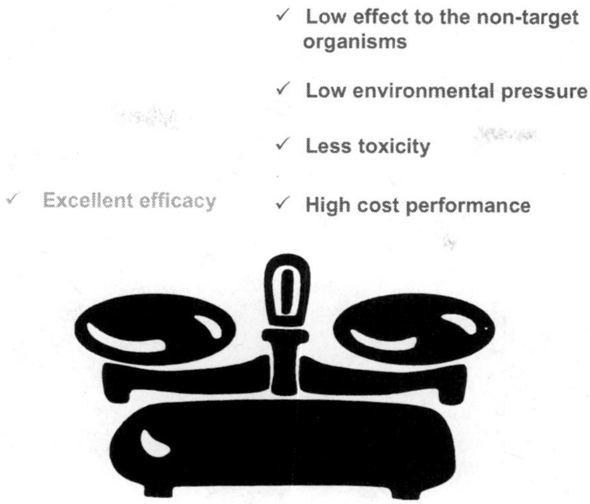

Figure 1. We have to balance all the requirements for the development of new insecticides.

Then, what is needed for the development of a new insecticide? Currently, the probability of inventing a new insecticide is 1 in 100,000, i.e., 100,000 useless chemicals are synthesized before one beneficial insecticide is invented. The probability of invention was 100 times greater 60 years ago during the brilliant age of organochloride and organophosphate insecticides. Development cost for one new insecticide is more than 100 million dollars. The development cost has increased exponentially over the past 60 years, mainly because of the increase in toxicological data requirements. This increase has been mainly due to the introduction of Good Laboratory Practice (GLP) and international harmonization concerning toxicological data requirements. Nearly 10 years are required for the development of a single new insecticide. Thousands of chemicals are synthesized and biologically screened every week. This screening process is a very fundamental and essential process but is also very monotonous and tedious. If we can obtain one or two candidate chemicals, they are subjected to the next step, including small-scale field trial, preliminary toxicological study, patent application, trial calculation of manufacturing cost, and formulation study. Two or three years are spent on this step. Moreover, no chemical can pass this step even if it fails to satisfy a single criterion in the requirement checklist. Now, we have a single chemical that has fulfilled all the criteria of the second step and can proceed to the next step. We begin to prepare a package consisting of toxicological study data and large-scale field test data that are required for registration to authorities such as the United States Environmental Protection Agency (USEPA). A minimum of 3–5 years are required for this step. Finally, we can submit the entire data package to the concerned authority. After submission, our documents are filed and frequently left unattended until registration 1 or more years later. Thus, it is evident that developing an insecticide is extremely expensive and laborious. It is, therefore, our duty to use insecticides in the most effective and prudent manner possible in order to maintain their effectiveness and sustain their use.

Insecticides for mosquito control

The most exciting event in the history of mosquito control was the invention of dichloro-diphenyl-trichloroethane (DDT) by Dr. Muller, who received the Nobel Prize for chemistry in 1948. The long persistence and excellent killing efficacy of DDT are responsible for its brilliant success after the Second World War. Nevertheless, the first DDT resistance case in *Anopheles* mosquitoes was detected several years later. Furthermore, DDT resistance was responsible for the increase in the incidence of malaria in the 1960s (*1*). Due to the failure of the malaria eradication program, the World Health Organization (WHO) has altered their policy from eradication to control. They recommend primary health care and the use of insecticide-impregnated mosquito nets. Olyset® Net is one of the most promising and long lasting insecticide-treated net (LLITN) (*2*). Olyset® Net is composed of plastic fibers impregnated with permethrin—one of the most popular and safe pyrethroids. Nowadays, pyrethroids are emerging as the predominant insecticides for vector control. They are used in various formulations such as in bed nets for the prevention of mosquito bites in malaria endemic areas, in ultra-low volume (ULV) sprays for emergency control of dengue vectors, and in space sprays in aircrafts and ships for the control of invading mosquitoes. In fact, pyrethroids comprise 40% of the insecticides used annually on a global level for indoor residual spraying against malaria vectors

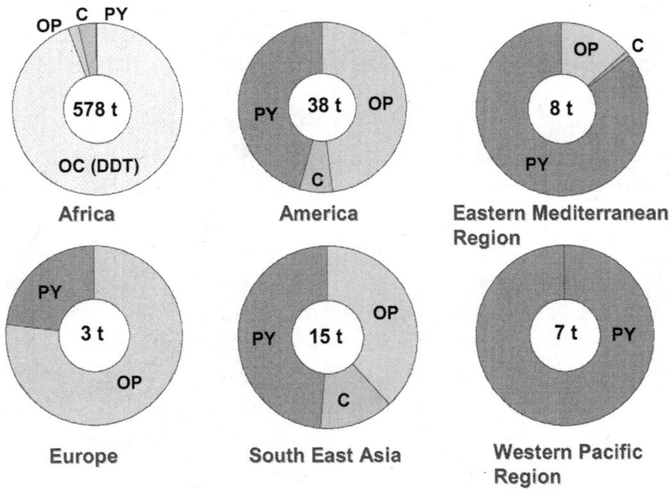

Figure 2*. Insecticide use for malaria vector control (Residual Spray, 2003-2005). OC, organochloride; OP, organophosphate; C, carbamate; PY, pyrethroid (Data obtained from reference 3)*

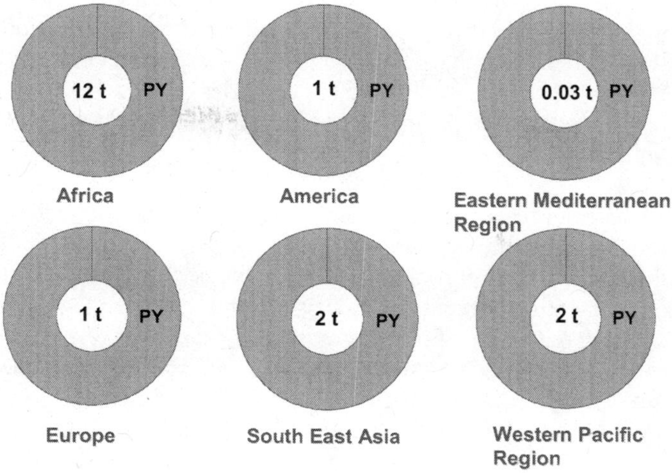

Figure 3. *Insecticide use for malaria vector control (Insecticide treated net, 2003-2005). OC, organochloride; OP, organophosphate; C, carbamate; PY, pyrethroid (Data obtained from reference 3)*

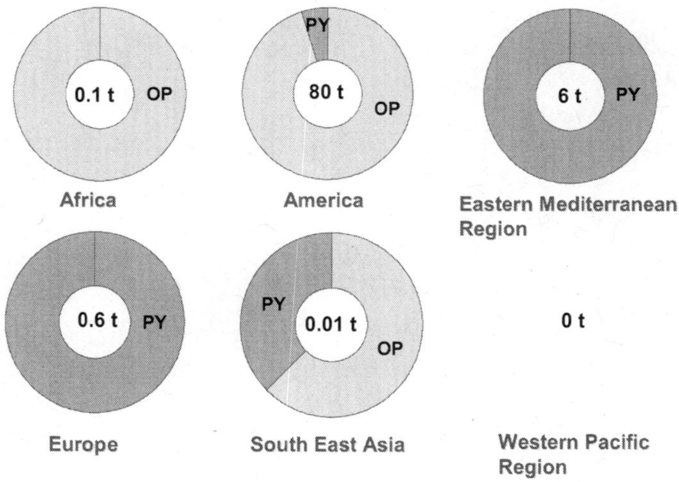

Figure 4. *Insecticide use for malaria vector control (Space spray, 2003-2005). OC, organochloride; OP, organophosphate; C, carbamate; PY, pyrethroid (Data obtained from reference 3)*

(Figure 2) and 100% of the WHO-recommended insecticides for the treatment of mosquito nets (Figure 3). The exception is the use of DDT in African countries (*3*). Organophosphates, as a space spraying formulation, are still taking major part in African, and Central and South American countries, but pyrethroids take a leading part in the other countries (Figure 4) (*3*).

What is pyrethroid?

Developmental research on pesticides of natural origin is believed to be a biorational approach since it may reduce the adverse environmental impact of chemicals on naturally occurring substances. One of the most successful events in the development of pesticide chemicals was the discovery of pyrethrum and the successful synthesis of pyrethroids. For example, classical synthetic pyrethroid allethrin (*4*) continues to be used for preventing mosquito bites without any toxicological and operational problems. The use of pyrethroids for preventing mosquito bites is believed to be biorational because this chemical is safe for mammals. Further, due to the low selection pressure of pyrethroids mosquitoes may develop minimum physiological resistance. Pyrethroid is the general term for a group of chemicals that includes natural pyrethrins derived from Chrysanthemum flowers and structurally related synthetic chemicals. Most of pyrethroids are highly nontoxic to mammals. Pyrethroids possess high

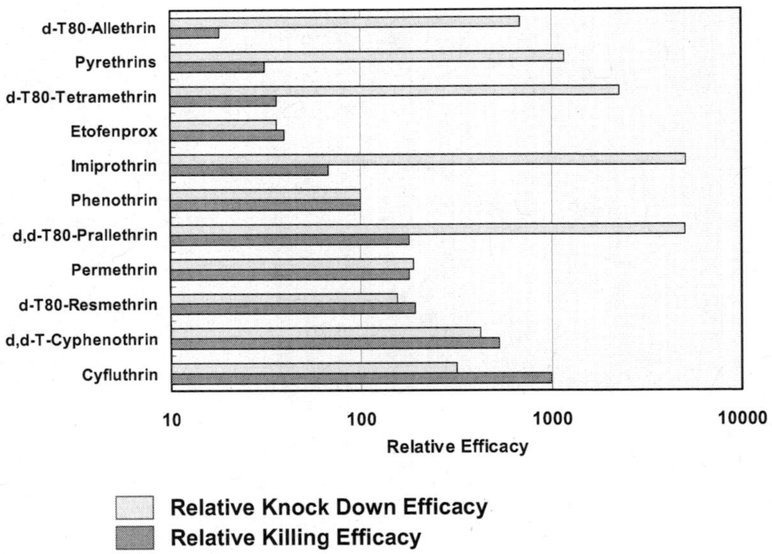

Figure 5. *Relative efficacy of pyrethroids against female Culex pipiens pallens.*

knockdown activity. Knockdown activity refers to fast-acting paralytic action that renders insects incapable of flying and disorients them (*5,6,7*). At present, pyrethroids account for more than 70% of household insecticides. Sodium channels located on axonal membranes are the primary targets of pyrethroids. The binding of pyrethroids and the consequent formation of binding contacts across different channel elements stabilize the channel in an open state, resulting in prolonged sodium tail currents (*8*). Recently, Sugiura and others (*9*) have found that after aerial spraying, most pyrethroid particles enter the insects' bodies via their spiracles and directly reach the central nervous system. There are two main groups of pyrethroids: one possessing high knockdown activity but low killing activity, and the other possessing high killing activity (Figure 5). The pyrethroids in the former group are aptly labeled as knockdown agents, and those in the latter group, as killing agents. Most of the pyrethroids belonging to the knockdown agent group contain a cyclopentenolone or an *N*-methylol or a related alcohol moiety. On the other hand, most pyrethroids belonging to the killing agent group contain a phenoxybenzyl alcohol or related alcohol moiety. Generally, the pyrethroids belonging to the latter group exhibit high photostability, which enables their outdoor use, for example, as agricultural pesticides.

Pyrethroids as ideal spatial repellents

The most popular and long-standing formulations using pyrethroids are mosquito coils, mosquito mats, and liquid vaporizers. Pyrethroids belonging to the knockdown agent group, such as allethrin, pyrethrin, and prallethrin, are used in these formulations. In particular, *d*-allethrin still continues to be used in these types of formulations. Further, mosquitoes have developed minimum physiological resistance to these pyrethroids due to the low selection pressure and low stability in the environment. In mosquito coils, the active ingredient is vaporized by heating the substrate by igniting the tip of mosquito coils. The optimum temperature of the portion undergoing vaporization is approximately 250°C. A heater equipped with a mosquito mat is heated at 150–160°C. The mechanism of a liquid vaporizer is slightly complicated, involving a ring-form heater, a wick for pumping up the liquid, and a bottle of pyrethroid solution.

Pyrethroids belonging to the knockdown agent group have been successfully used worldwide for a long period. Recently, a group of newly developed pyrethroids with high vapor pressure has come to open new era for pyrethroids. Metofluthrin, one of the above promising pyrethroids, is newly synthesized and produced by Sumitomo Chemical Co. Ltd., Osaka, Japan; having high insecticidal activity and high vapor pressure (*10*). Metofluthrin belongs to the group of knockdown agents but has a unique characteristic of high vapor pressure. The vapor pressure of Metofluthrin is >2 times and >100 times higher than that of *d*-allethrin and permethrin, respectively, and it vaporizes at room temperature without heating, while other conventional pyrethroids require heating for vaporization. Another unique characteristic is its high efficacy against mosquitoes which is 28–79 times more effective than *d*-allethrin (*11*). These unique characteristics of Metofluthrin may lead to the development of new mosquito controlling devices that do not require any external energy for vaporization and have low cost and longer effective duration. Numerous field trials in residential houses have assessed the effectiveness of Metofluthrin-impregnated plastic strips against dengue and malaria vectors (*12,13,14,15,16,17*).

Here, we define the term "spatial repellency". Spatial repellency is classified into 2 categories. One is "directional repellency" wherein insects are physically repelled from the area but retain their directionality (*18*). The other is "non-directional repellency" wherein insects lose their directionality (*19*). In the latter case, only some insects are repelled from the area; however, the insects that are not repelled are nevertheless physiologically affected; they are either knocked down or

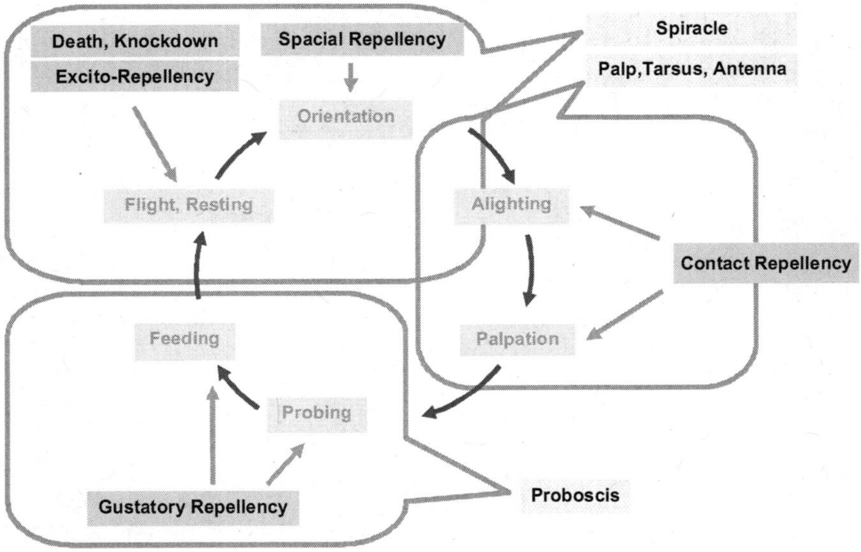

Figure 6. The sequence of mosquito activities with possible points of pyrethroid effects. (modified from reference 20)

their orientation towards the host is disturbed. Spatial repellency of pyrethroids appears to belong to the latter category. Spatial repellency is considered to occur through two main modes of pyrethroid action: knockdown activity and biting inhibition or disruption of orientation toward the host (excito-repellency). The principal mode of entry of the repellent is thought to be through the spiracles (Figure 6). Excito-repellency may be categorized as a sublethal mode that results from neural excitement, which appears to occur at an earlier stage of toxication or with a dosage that is lower than that required for knockdown or death (*7*). Winney (*6*) reported that female *Aedes aegypti* exposed for a few minutes to the smoke of a pyrethroid-based mosquito coil did not bite. MacIver (*5*) defined the "repellency" associated with pyrethroids as a reaction of mosquitoes at the threshold level when the neural activation and knockdown occur, resulting in the loss of power to orient toward their hosts. Such spatial repellency will not induce any pyrethroid resistance since it does not kill the affected insects and causes no selection pressure on insect populations.

Pyrethroid as double-edged sword

As explained in the previous section, the discovery of the phenoxybenzyl alcohol moiety accelerated the development of photo-stable pyrethroids that could be used for outdoor use such as agricultural purposes. These "second generation" pyrethroids have been used worldwide as good vector control agents with various application techniques, such as residual spraying, ULV spraying, and bed net treatment (long-lasting insecticide-treated net [LLITN]). However, photo-stable and highly effective pyrethroids might accelerate the development of pyrethroid resistance in mosquito populations. Photo-stable pyrethroids persist on substrates such as wall and floor surfaces and continue to kill insects on contact for a long period. This induces a strong selection pressure on the insect population. Ultra-low volume (ULV) space sprays are commonly applied for the emergency control of dengue vectors in urban areas. Space sprays by themselves do not induce a very strong selection pressure; however, uncontrolled treatment at high frequency facilitates the development of resistance. In the past, the use of pyrethroids in aqueous environments was impossible since pyrethroids are highly toxic to aqueous organisms. However, recently, a new pyrethroid with low fish toxicity has been commercially produced and is widely used in aqueous environments such as paddy fields. This might cause considerable selection pressure on the mosquito larvae distributed in such environments. The most serious problem is that resistance to a single pyrethroid causes cross-resistance to all other pyrethroids, including knockdown agents. In fact, many reports concerning pyrethroid resistance have emerged after the successful application of pyrethroids as vector control agents (*21*). Cross-resistance to knockdown agents is the most serious problem.

Distribution analysis of pyrethroid resistance in the dengue vectors, *Aedes aegypti* and *Ae. albopictus* in Vietnam

Since the pyrethroid resistance in mosquitoes is a global phenomenon, we have started to monitor the distribution of mosquito resistance to pyrethroids. The first pilot study has been carried out in Vietnam since 2006 as a cooperative research with the National Institute of Hygiene and Epidemiology, Hanoi, Vietnam. In the course of the National Dengue Control Program in Vietnam, the ecological differences between two dengue vectors, namely, *Aedes aegypti* and *Ae. albopictus*, that are of different geographical origins, have become a subject of discussion. The ecological differences in the vectors may be the reason for the differences in the epidemics occurring nationwide. In order to examine a nationwide distribution of the two species and pyrethroid resistance, used tires, one of the main breeding grounds of the two species, were targeted for larval collection. Used tires were suitable as a standard container because they were extensively and commonly distributed along roads in Vietnam.

Collection of mosquito larvae from used tires and the simplified knockdown test using the larvae

We periodically drove along the national road from the north end to the Mekong Delta in Vietnam and collected mosquito larvae from used tires (Figure 7). Whenever we encountered the used tires, most of which were found along the periphery of repair shops (Figure 8), while driving along a systematically determined route, geographical position (with a global positioning system [GPS]), number of tires, presence of water in the tires, existence of mosquito larvae in the tires, and environmental characteristics such as land with vegetation within a 25-m radius; and distribution of houses along the road, were recorded. Mosquito larvae were collected from the tires with larvae (6-20 tires per site) by netting (5 times per tire). The collected larvae, except those used for the susceptibility test, were placed in 1.5 ml plastic vials containing ethanol solution for identification at a later time.

The most plausible procedures for investigating the knockdown susceptibility of mosquitoes to pyrethroids is to acquire an adequate number of field-collected female adults or laboratory-reared colonies by rearing field-collected larvae and to carry out a knockdown bioassay with the adults and the actual pyrethroid formulation, such as a mosquito coil, in a laboratory. However, it was impossible for us to follow this procedure since more than 180 field-collected larval colonies were acquired in the present study. Susceptibility tests were, therefore, performed on the day of collection according to a simplified protocol by using the fourth instar larvae (Figure 9). Each larva was placed in a glass vial with 20 ml of water. An emulsifiable concentrate of 90% *d*-T_{80}-allethrin was diluted with water to obtain a 250 ppm solution. After releasing the larva, 32 or 8 μl of the solution was poured in each vial to obtain a concentration of 0.4 and 0.1 ppm, respectively. Ten larvae from each site were used for each concentration regime. Knockdown of the larvae was observed for 30 min. After the test, each larva was placed in a 1.5 ml plastic vial containing ethanol solution for identification at a later time. After identification, individual knockdown data were summarized for each mosquito species (*Ae. aegypti*, *Ae. albopictus*, and *Culex quinquefasciatus*). The median knockdown times (KT_{50}s), i.e., the time required for 50% knockdown, were scored according to the 6 following categories: 1, <5 min; 2, 5-10 min; 3, 10-15 min; 4, 15-20 min; 5, 20-30 min; and 6, >30 min). The susceptibility index was calculated as the product of the scores at 0.1 and 0.4 ppm. Thus, a mosquito colony with a susceptibility index of 1 was considered to be the most susceptible and a colony with a susceptibility index of 36 was considered to be the least susceptible to *d*-allethrin. Multiple regression analysis was performed to analyze the effects of geographical, environmental, and social factors on susceptibility. Altitude and latitude at each collection point were used as the geographical and environmental factors, and province-based population density (persons per square kilometer) and the annual number of dengue fever cases in 2005 were used as the social factors. Additionally, annual province-based pyrethroid use for dengue vector control in

2007 and annual province-based pyrethroid use for malaria vector control in 1998-2007 were also used. Province-based data were transformed into a raster image using the spline function with ArcGIS 9.2 (ESRI Japan Corp.) to obtain extrapolated values at the collection points.

Figure 10 shows the correlation between the larval susceptibility index and adult KT_{50} of the same colony of *Ae. aegypti* for samples collected from several places in Vietnam. A relatively high correlations in knockdown susceptibility were observed between larvae and adults, indicating that the present simplified knockdown test is a good reflection of adult susceptibility.

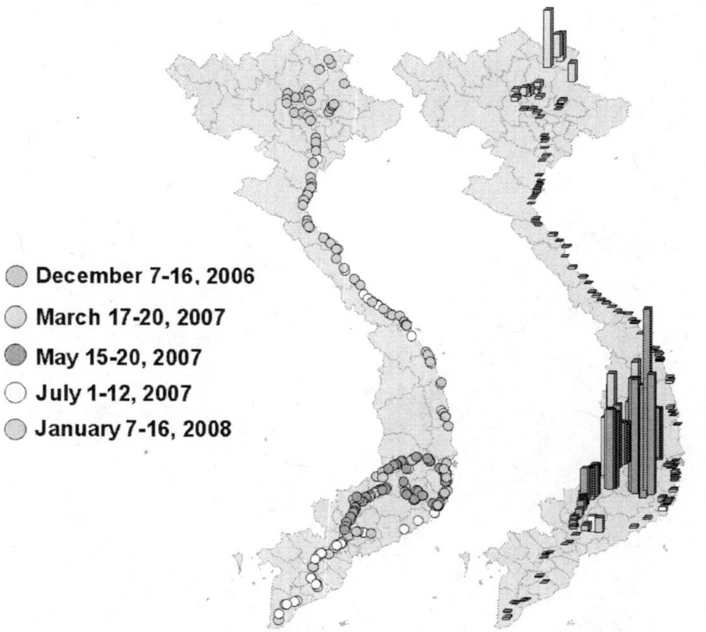

Figure 7. *The date and location of the mosquito collection from used tires in Vietnam. The bars in the right map indicate the relative altitude at each collection point (The highest bar indicates 1563 m). (Reproduced from reference 22).*
(See page 1 of color inserts.)

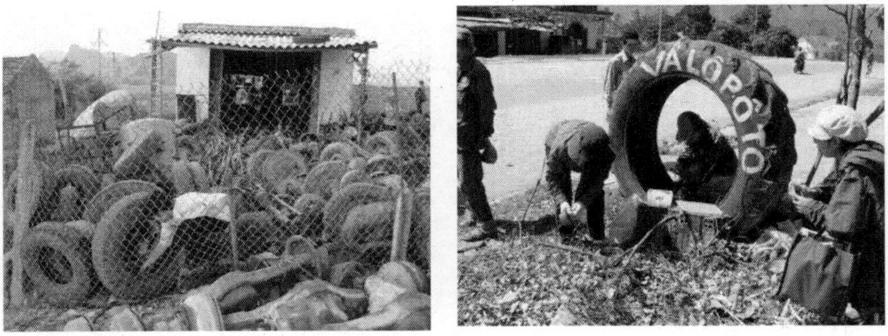

Figure 8. *Mosquito collection from used tires in Vietnam.*

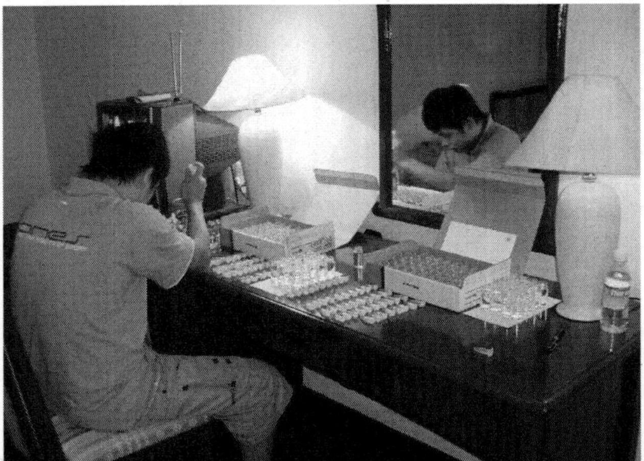

Figure 9. *Knockdown test using individual mosquito larva.*

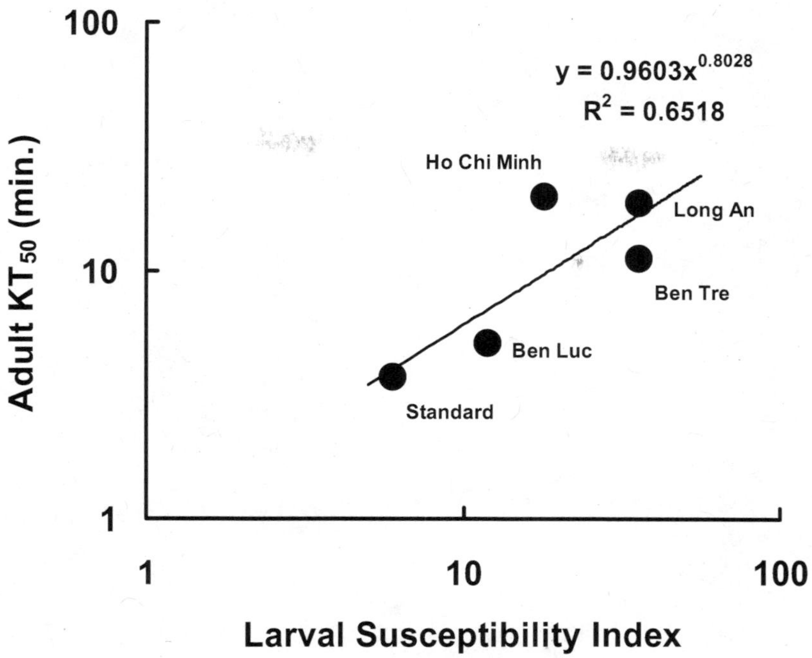

Figure 10. *Correlation between the larval susceptibility index and adult KT_{50} of Ae. aegypti collected from several places in Vietnam. Each plot indicates the location where a mosquito colony was collected. The adult KT_{50} was calculated by the knockdown test by burning 0.5 g of mosquito coil containing 0.3% (w/w) d-allethrin in a glass chamber (70 x 70 x 70 cm). (Reproduced from reference 22).*

Geographical distribution of mosquito species and susceptibility against *d*-allethrin in used tires in Vietnam

Larvae were collected from used tires along roads in Vietnam from 267 collection points throughout the first half of collection surveillance (7–16 December 2006; 17–20 March, 15–20 May). Used tires were extensively and commonly distributed. Collection sites were categorized into 5 areas: (1) northern mountainous area (172–506 m in height), (2) northern plain area, (3) eastern coastal area, (4) southern mountainous area (103–1563 m in height), and (5) southern wetlands. Among the total 21412 tires found in total during the first half of investigation from December 2006 to may 2007, 2141 were examined and 1554 contained water (72.6%); 484 contained mosquitoes (31.1%) and of these, 333 contained dengue vector mosquitoes (*Ae. aegypti* and *Ae. albopictus*) (21.4%). In total, 3887 *Ae. aegypti*, 3039 *Ae. albopictus*, and 7005 *Cx.*

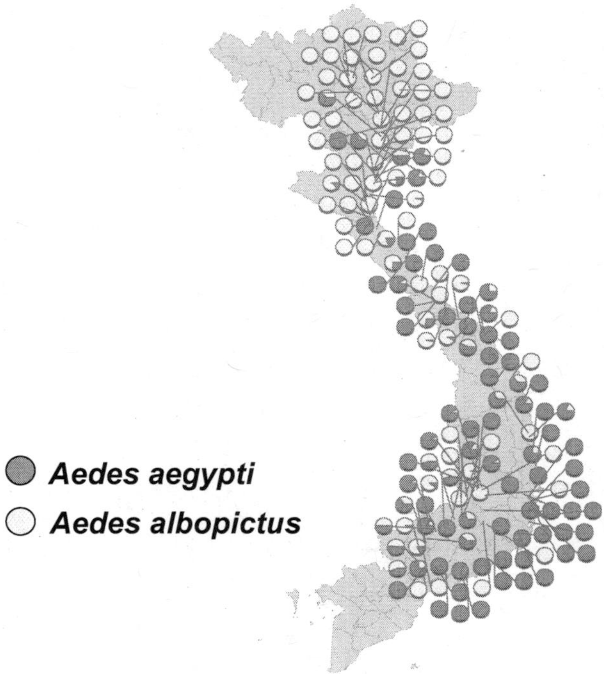

Figure 11. *Species composition of mosquito larvae collected from used tires in Vietnam. (Reproduced from reference 23)*
(See page 1 of color inserts.)

quinquefasciatus larvae were collected. In the northern part of Vietnam, *Ae. albopictus* was dominant, and this dominance gradually reduced toward the south. *Ae. aegypti* was dominant in the southern part. In the eastern coastal areas of the southern part, almost 100% of the *Aedes* larvae collected were *Ae. aegypti*. However, in the mountainous areas, the number of *Ae. albopictus* increased, suggesting that the distribution of the two species is determined by different environmental gradients (Figure 11) (*23*).

Susceptibility indices for *Ae. aegypti*, *Ae. albopictus*, and *Cx. quinquefasciatus* are shown in Figure 12. The number of points where the susceptibility tests were carried out were 67 for *Ae. aegypti*, 50 for *Ae. albopictus*, and 73 for *Cx. quinquefasciatus*. The average susceptibility index and the proportion of mosquito colonies with susceptibility indices greater than 20 was 24.9 and 59.7% for *Ae. aegypti*, 8.48 and 8.0% for *Ae. albopictus*, and 12.6 and 21.9% for *Cx. quinquefasciatus*, respectively (*22*). When compared with the other species, reduction in susceptibility was most prominent in *Ae. aegypti*. In contrast, the reduction in the susceptibility of *Ae. albopictus* and *Cx. quinquefasciatus* was moderate. The susceptibility of the abovementioned species to *d*-allethrin was lower in the southern part than in the northern part of

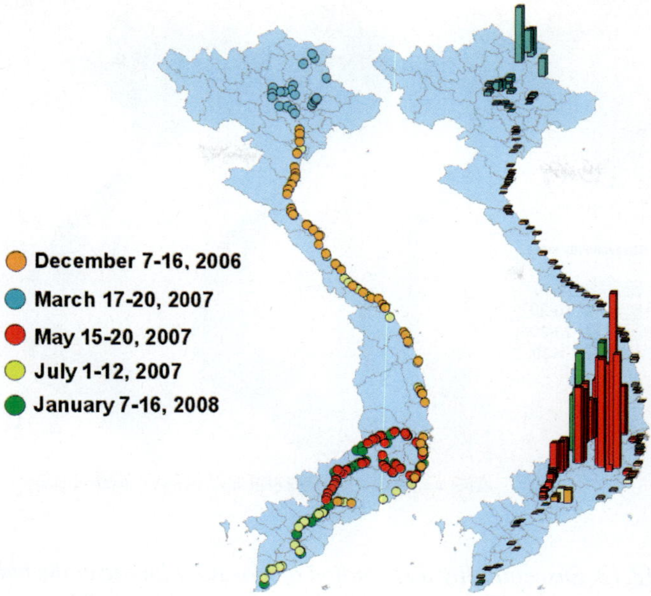

Figure 13.7. The date and location of the mosquito collection from used tires in Vietnam. The bars in the right map indicate the relative altitude at each collection point (The highest bar indicates 1563 m). (Reproduced from reference 22).

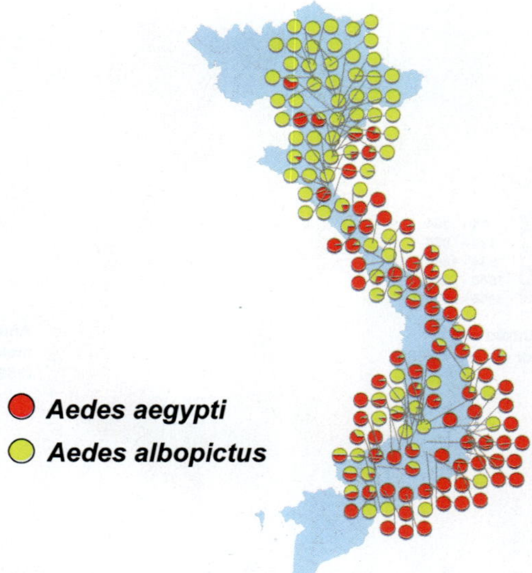

Figure 13.11. Species composition of mosquito larvae collected from used tires in Vietnam. (Reproduced from reference 23)

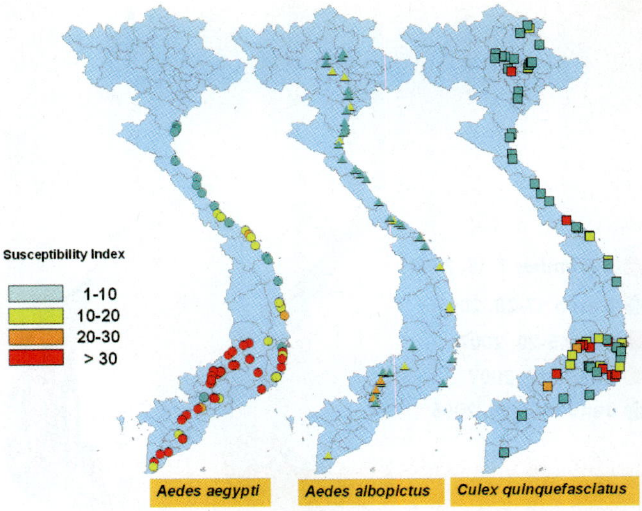

Figure 13.12. Susceptibility distribution of mosquito larvae collected in used tires in Vietnam. (Reproduced from reference 22)

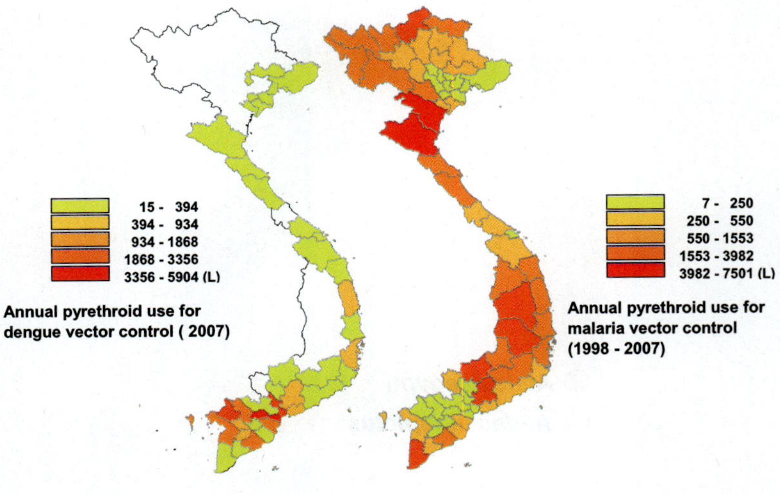

Figure 13.13. Annual pyrethroid use for dengue and malaria vector control in Vietnam. The blanks in the map indicate that no data were available (Reproduced from reference 22).

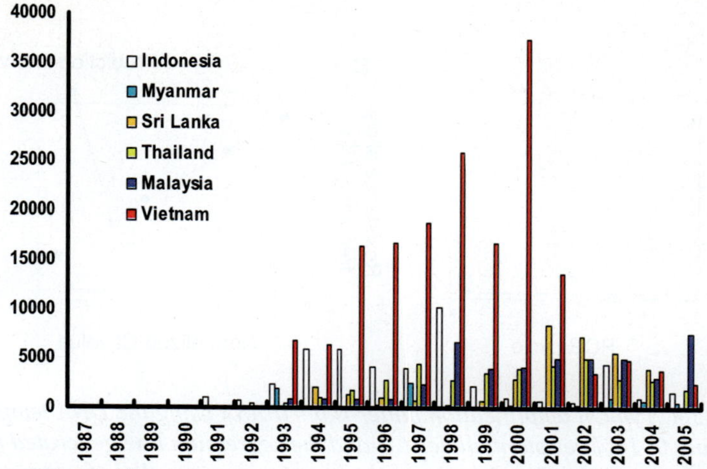

Figure 13.14. Change in the annual use of pyrethroids (kg as active ingredient) for malaria control in South East Asian countries. (Data obtained from reference 3)

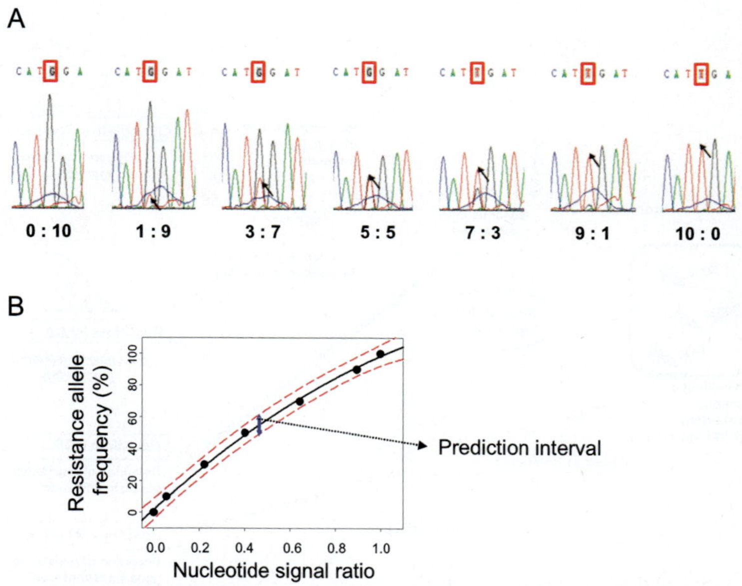

Figure 15.1. Sequencing chromatograms of the standard template DNA mixtures with different ratios of resistant and susceptible alleles (A) and the plot of resistance sequence signal ratio versus resistance allele frequency at the M815I mutation site (B). The relative intensities of the resistance allele signals are indicated with arrows in Panel A. Quadratic regression line is indicated by a solid line with the upper and lower 95% prediction lines indicated by dotted lines in Panel B.

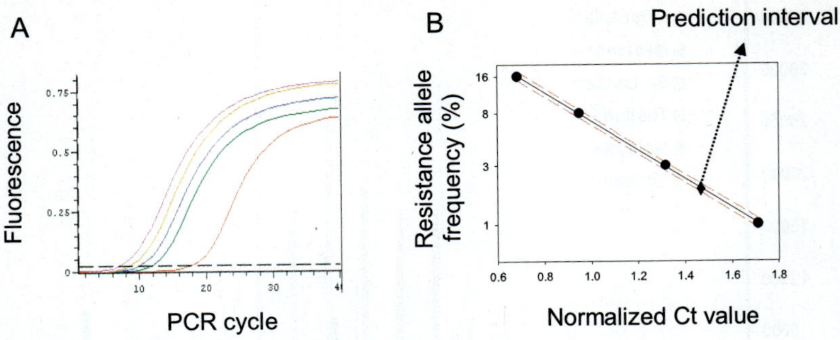

Figure 15.4. Typical amplification patterns of rtPASA using the DNA templates containing 0~16% resistant alleles (A) and the regression line generated from the plot of normalized Ct value versus the log of resistance allele frequency (B). The regression line is indicated by a solid line with the upper and lower 95% prediction lines indicated by dotted lines in Panel B

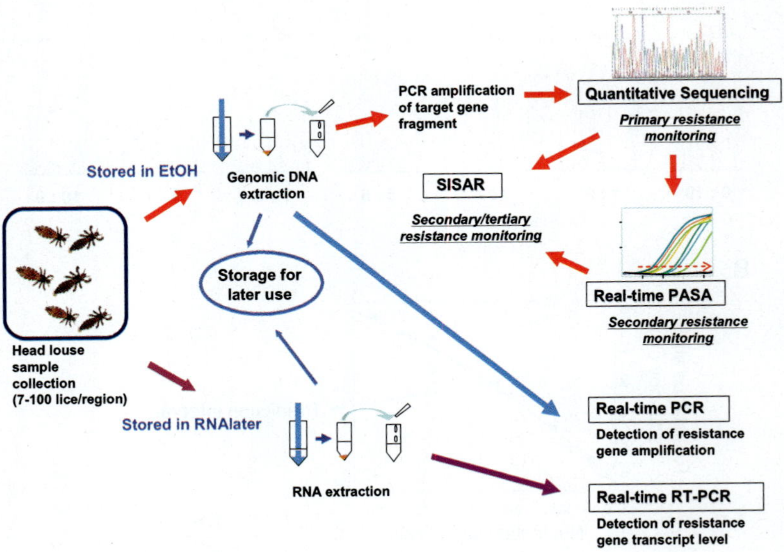

Figure 15.6. Schematic diagram of head lice resistance monitoring tire using several molecular tools.

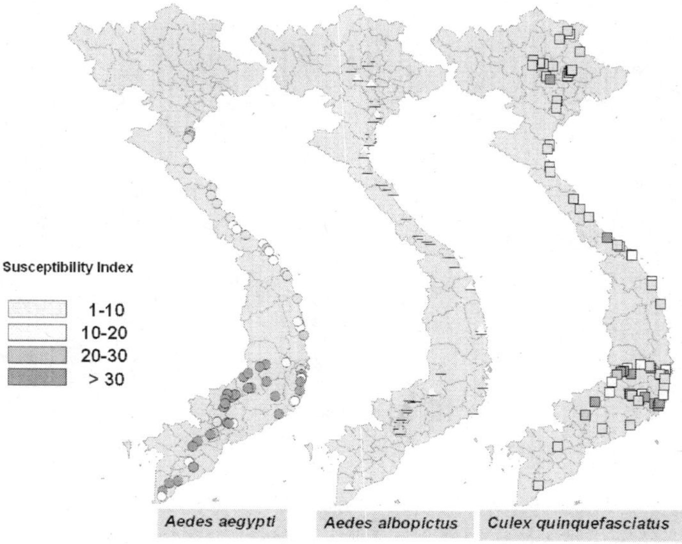

Figure 12. *Susceptibility distribution of mosquito larvae collected in used tires in Vietnam. (Reproduced from reference 22) (See page 2 of color inserts.)*

Vietnam. For *Ae. aegypti*, multiple regression analysis showed significant increases in the susceptibility indices with decrease in the latitude of the collection points. There was, however, no significant correlation between the susceptibility indices and population density, annual number of dengue cases, and annual pyrethroid use for dengue control for *Ae. aegypti* and *Ae. albopictus* (*22*). The only exception in both species was the significant correlation between the susceptibility indices and the annual pyrethroid use for malaria control in *Ae. aegypti* (*22*).

One hypothetical reason for the above might be that treatment with large amounts of pyrethroids was concentrated in the southern part of Vietnam for dengue vector control and not in the northern part since dengue fever is more prevalent in the southern part. However, the correlations between the susceptible indices and annual number of dengue cases or annual pyrethroid use for dengue vector control in *Ae. aegypti* and *Ae. albopictus* were not significant, indicating the existence of another factor. Another reason might be the use of DDT and pyrethroids as residual treatment inside houses and pyrethroid-impregnated bed nets for malaria control that were used nationwide as a part of the National Malaria Control Program (Figure 13) (*24,25,26*). The latter explanation seems to be more plausible since *Ae. aegypti* demonstrated remarkably low susceptibility in highland areas where forest malaria continues to be endemic (*27,28,29*). The high correlation between the susceptibility indices and the annual pyrethroid use for malaria vector control in *Ae. aegypti* might support the above explanation (Table 1). In Vietnam, 24 tones of DDT was used for residual treatment against

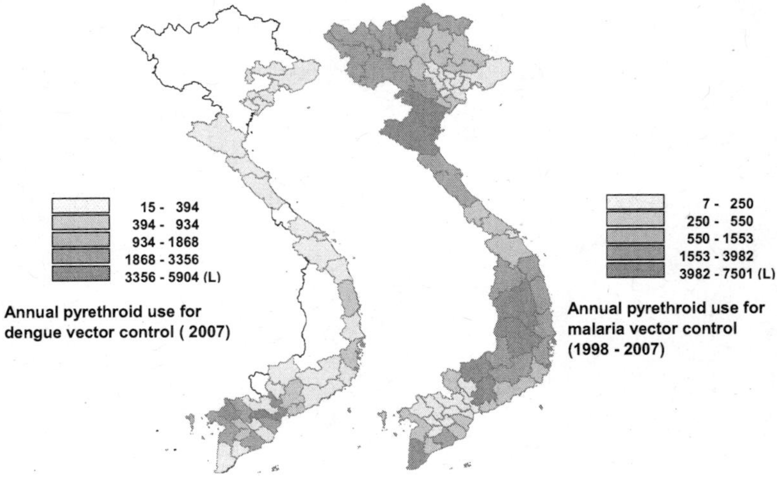

Figure 13. *Annual pyrethroid use for dengue and malaria vector control in Vietnam. The blanks in the map indicate that no data were available (Reproduced from reference 22).*
(See page 2 of color inserts.)

malaria vectors in 1993 and 1994. However, since the abandoning of DDT sprays in 1995, only pyrethroids (spraying of λ-cyhalothrin and occasionally deltamethrin, and permethrin-impregnated bed nets) have been extensively used in large amounts in Vietnam, unlike in the other Asian countries (Figure 14) (*3,26*). The abovementioned insecticide treatment appears to have been intensively conducted in the interior and along the periphery of human habitation

Table I. Stepwise multiple regression analysis for determination of correlation between the susceptibility indices of mosquitoes and geographical and social factors

Factor	*Aedes aegypti*		*Aedes albopictus*	
	Estimated Value	*p*	Estimated Value	*p*
Latitude	-1.14	0.0001	-	-
Altitude (m)	-	-	-	-
Population density	-	-	-	-
Annual dengue cases (2005)	-	-	-	-
Annual pyrethroid use for dengue vector control (2007)	-	-	-	-
Annual pyrethroid use for malaria vector control (1998-2007)	1.65	0.0028	-	-

(Reproduced from reference 22)

areas, where incidentally the breeding and resting sites of *Ae. aegypti* are located. This might account for the strong selection pressure against *Ae. aegypti* and not so much against *Ae. albopictus* since Asian *Ae. aegypti* is generally a domestic and endophagic that has a greater preference for indoor breeding than *Ae. albopictus* (*30,31,32,33,34*). Several papers report the pyrethroid resistance of both Asian *Ae. aegypti* and *Ae. albopictus*. Most of them report that *Ae. aegypti* had higher pyrethroid resistance than *Ae. albopictus*, indicating pyrethroid resistance was affected by ecological differences in mosquitoes (*35,36,37,38*).

Although details regarding the amount of insecticides used for dengue vector control in Vietnam have not been published, 21,000 liters of photo-stable pyrethroid formulations such as α-cyhalothrin, deltamethrin, and permethrin was reported to be used for dengue vector control in 20 southern provinces in 2007 (personal communication). The extensive use of photo-stable pyrethroids, therefore, seems to have been very common in Vietnam.

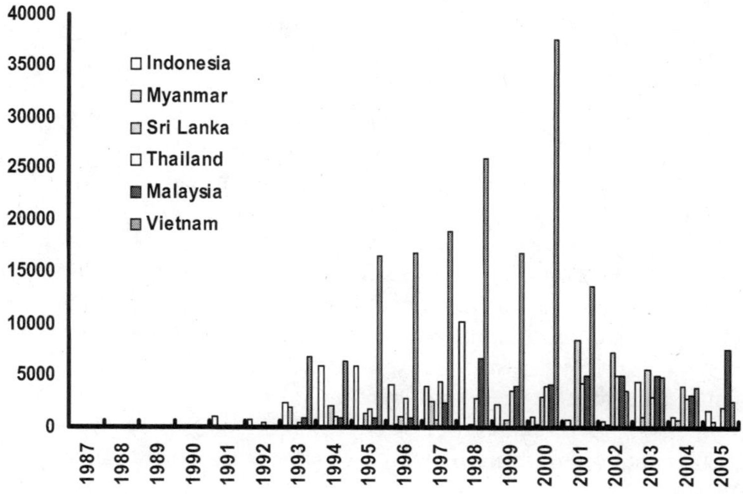

Figure 14. *Change in the annual use of pyrethroids (kg as active ingredient) for malaria control in South East Asian countries. (Data obtained from reference 3) (See page 3 of color inserts.)*

Conclusion

Insecticides still provide the most promising countermeasures for controlling malaria, dengue hemorrhagic fever (DHF), and other arthropod-borne diseases. On an average, at the global level, 547 tones of DDT, 39 tones of organophosphates, 23 tones of carbamates, and 41 tones of pyrethroids are used as active ingredients annually for indoor residual spraying against malaria vectors (*3*). The average total amount of pyrethroids used annually as active ingredients between 2003 and 2005 at the global level was 161 tones, which is 16% of the total insecticide consumption and 36% of the total insecticide consumption if the amount of DDT, which is exclusively used in African countries, is excluded. Among pyrethroids that are used for vector control, 98.7% comprise photo-stable pyrethroids such as α-cypermethrin, bifenthrin, cyfluthrin, cypermethrin, deltamethrin, etofenprox, λ-cyhalothrin, and permethrin (*3*). Pyrethroid resistance will be a major problem for the vector control program since at present, there are no suitable chemical substitutes for pyrethroids. In order to effectively manage pyrethroid resistance, the establishment of a feasible insecticide management system and a regular monitoring system of insecticide susceptibility will be essential. Moreover, it is expected that the use of photo-unstable knockdown agents as spatial repellents, which effectively interfere with disease transmission without causing any selection pressure to insect populations, will be reconsidered.

Acknowledgment

We thank D. T. Trinh, National Institute of Malariology, Parasitology and Entomology, Hanoi, Vietnam, T. V. Phong, National Institute of Hygiene and Epidemiology, Hanoi, Vietnam, T. T. T. Huynh and L. L. Luu, Pasteur Institute, Ho Chi Minh city, Vietnam, C. Tsurukawa and T. Abe, Institute of Tropical Medicine, Nagasaki University, Nagasaki, Japan, T. Otaguro and N. Takamura, School of Medicine, Nagasaki University, Nagasaki, Japan, and Y. Kuroda, K. Misaki, , N. Ukishiro, and Y. Sakata, Sumika Techno-Service Co., Ltd., Hyogo, Japan, for their technical support, rearing and providing the experimental insects, and assisting in this study. This study is supported by Core University Program sponsored and Grant-in-Aid for Scientific Research by the Japan Society for the Promotion of Science (JSPS) and the Collaborative Study on Emerging and Re-emerging Infectious Diseases in Vietnam: Enhancement of Research Capacity.

References

1. Bruce-Chwatt, L. J. *Essential Malariology*; John Wiley & Sons: New York, 1985.
2. *Report of the 5th WHOPES Working Group meeting*, World Health Organization, 2001.
3. Zaim, M.; Jambulingam, P. *Globalinsecticide use for vector-borne disease control*, World Health Organization, 2007.
4. Schechter, M. S.; Green, N.; Laforge, F. B. 1949. *Journal American Chemical Society*, 1949, *71*, 3165-3173.
5. MacIver, D. R. *Pyrethrum Post* **1964,** *7*, 7-14.
6. Winney, R. *Pyrethrum Post* **1975,** *13,* 17-22.
7. Birley, M. H.; Mutero, C. M.; Turner, I. F.; Chadwick, P. R. *Annals of Tropical Medicine and Parasitology* **1987,** *81*, 163-171.

8. O'Reilly, A. O.; Khambay, B. P.; Williamson, M. S.; Field, L. M.; Wallace, B. A.; Davies, T. G. *Biochemical Journal* **2006,** *396*, 255-263.
9. Sugiura, M; Horibe, Y.; Kawada, H.; Takagi, M. *Insecticide Biochemistry and Physiology,* **2008,** 91, 135-140.
10. Ujihara, K.; Mori, T.; Iwasaki, T.; Sugano, M.; Shono, Y.; Matsuo, N. *Bioscience,Biotechnology,and Biochemistry* **2004,** *68*, 170-174.
11. Argueta, T. B. O.; Kawada, H.: Sugano, M.; Kubota, S.; Shono, Y.; Tsushima, K.; Takagi, M. *Medical Entomology and Zoology* **2004,** *55*, 211-216.
12. Kawada, H.; Maekawa, Y.; Tsuda, Y.; Takagi, M. *Journal of American Mosquito Control Association* **2004,** *20,* 292-298.
13. Kawada, H.; Maekawa, Y.; Tsuda, Y.; Takagi, M. *Journal of American Mosquito Control Association* **2004,** *20,* 434-437.
14. Kawada, H.; Nguyen T. Y.; Nguyen T. H.; Trang M. S.; Nguyen V. D.; Takagi, M. *American Journal of Tropical Medicine and Hygiene* **2005,** *73,* 350-353.
15. Kawada, H.; Maekawa, Y.; Takagi, M. *Journal of Vector Ecology* 2005, *30,* 181-185.
16. Kawada, H.; Iwasaki, T.; Lu, L. L. Tran, K. T.; Nguyen, T. N. M.; Shono, Y. ; Katayama, Y; Takagi, M. *American Journal of Tropical Medicine and Hygiene* **2006,** *75,* 1153-1157.
17. Kawada, H.; Temu, E. A. Minjas, J. N.; Matsumoto, O.; Iwasaki, T.; Takagi, M. *Journal of American Mosquito Control Association* **2008,** *in press.*
18. Dethier, V. G.; Browne, L. B.; Smith, C. N. *Journal of Economic Entomology* **1960,** *53,* 134-136.
19. Kennedy, J. S. *Bulletin of Entomological research* **1947,** *37,* 593-607.
20. Chadwick, P. R. *Mosquito News* **1970,** *30,* 162-170.
21. African Network for Vector Resistance. *WHO* 2005.
22. Kawada, H.; Higa, Y.; Nguyen, T. Y.; Tran H. S.; Nguyen, T. H.; Takagi, M. *PLoS Neglected Tropical Diseases* **2008,** *in review.*
23. Higa, Y.; Nguyen, T. Y.; Kawada, H.; Tran, H. S.; Nguyen T. H.; Takagi, M. *Unpublished.*
24. Verlé, P.; Lieu, T. T. T.; Kongs, A., der Stuyft, P. V.; Coosemans, M. *Tropical Medicine and International Health* **1999**, *4,* 139-145.
25. Hung, L. Q.; de Vries, P. J.; Giao, P. T.; Nam, N. V.; Binh, T. Q.; Chong, M. T.; Quoc, N. T. T. A.; Thanh, T. N.; Hung, L. N.; Kager, P. A. *Bulletin of World Health Organization* **2002**, *80*, 660-666.
26. Nam, N. V.; de Vries, P. J.; Toi, L. V.; Nagelkerke, N. *Tropical Medicine and International Health* **2005**, *10,* 357-365.
27. Erhart, A.; Thang, N. D.; Hung, N. Q.; Toi, L. V.; Hung, L. X.; Tuy, T. Q.; Cong, L. D.; Speybroecck, N.; Coosemans, M.; D'Alessandro, U. *American Journal of Tropical Medicine and Hygiene* **2004**, *70*, 110–118.
28. Erhart, A.; Thang, N. D.; Ky, P. V.; Tinh, T. T.; Overmeir1, C. V.; Speybroeck1, N.; Obsomer, V.; Hung, L. X.; Thuan, L. K.; Coosemans1, M.; D'alessandro1, U. *Malaria Journal* **2005**, *4*, 58.
29. Thang, N. D.; Erhart, A.; Speybroeck, N.; Hung, L. X.; Thuan, L. K.; Hung, C. T.; Ky, P. V.; Coosemans, M.; D'Alessandro, U. *Malaria Journal* **2008**, *7*, 28.

30. Hawley, W. A. *Journal of American Mosquito Control Association* **1988**., *4 (Suppl. 1)*, 1-39.
31. Edman, J. E.; Kittayapong, P.; Linthicum, K.; Scott, T. Journal of American Mosquito Control Association **1997**, *13*, 24–27.
32. Ishak, H.; Miyagi, I.; Toma, T.; Kamimura, K. *Southeast Asian Journal of Tropical Medicine and Public Health* **1997**, *28*, 844–850.
33. Higa, Y.; Tsuda, Y.; Tuno, N.; Takagi, M. *Medical Entomology and Zoology* **2001**, *52*, 105–116.
34. Tsuda, Y.; Suwonkerd, W.; Chawprom, S.; Prajakwong, S.; Takagi, M. *Journal of American Mosquito Control Association* **2006**, *22*, 222–228.
35. Ping, L. T.; Yatiman, R.; Gek, L. S. *Journal of American Mosquito Control Association* **2001**, *17*, 144-146.
36. Ponlawat, A.; Scott, J. G.; Harrington, L. C. Insecticide Susceptibility of Aedes aegypti and Aedes albopictus across Thailand. J. Med. Entomol. 2005.42:821-825.
37. Jirakanjanakit, N.; Rongnoparut, P.; Saengtharatip, S.; Chareonviriyaphap, T.; Duchon, S.; Bellec, C.; Yoksani, S. *Journal of Economic Entomology* **2007**, *100*, 545-550.
38. Pethuan, S.; Jirakanjanakit, N.; Saengtharatip, S.; Chareonviriyaphap, T.; Kaewpa, D.; Rongnoparut, P. *Tropical Biomedicine* **2007**, *24*,7–15.

Chapter 14

The Body Louse, *Pediculus humanus humanus* (Phthiraptera: Pediculidae), Genome Project: Past, Present, and Opportunities for the Future

Barry R. Pittendrigh[1], J. M. Clark[2], S. H. Lee[3], W. Sun[1], and E. Kirkness[4]

[1]Department of Entomology, University of Illinois at Urbana-Champaign, Urbana, IL 61801
[2]Department of Veterinary and Animal Science, University of Massachusetts, Amherst, MA 01003
[3]Department of Agricultural Biotechnology, Seoul National University, Seoul, South Korea
[4]J. Craig Venter Institute, 9704 Medical Center Drive, Rockville, MD 20850

The human body louse, *Pediculus humanus humanus* (L.) and the human head louse, *P. humanus capitis,* belong to the hemimetabolous order Phthiraptera. The body louse is the primary vector that transmits the bacterial agents of louse-borne relapsing fever, trench fever, and epidemic typhus. The genomes of the bacterial causative agents of several of these aforementioned diseases have been sequenced. Thus, determining the body louse genome will enhance studies of host-vector-pathogen interactions. Although not important as a major disease vector, head lice are of major social concern. Resistance has developed to traditional pesticides used to control head and body lice. It is imperative that new molecular targets be discovered for the development of novel compounds to control these insects. No complete genome sequence yet exists for a hemimetabolous insect species. In large part, this is because hemimetabolous insects often have large (2,000 MB) to very large (up to 16,300 MB) genomes. Fortuitously, we determined that the human body louse has one of the smallest genome sizes known in the insect world, making it a suitable choice as a minimal hemimetabolous genome in which many genes have been eliminated during its adaptation to human parasitism. Since many lice species infest birds and mammals, the body louse genome-sequencing project will facilitate studies of their comparative genomics. Recently, the body louse genome has been sequenced and the Body Louse Genome Consortium (BLGC) is currently annotating the genome. Questions that will be addressed by the BLGC are outlined in the following article. We also raise possible future directions for research on body lice.

Lice are species-specific parasites and phylogenetic evidence suggests that chimpanzees and human lice diverged about 5.6 million years ago, the same time since these two mammalian species shared a common ancestor (*1*). Body lice, *Pediculus humanus humanus* (L.) live in close contact with humans and are often spread by shared bedding or by close personal contact (*2*). This pest typically lives in the seams of the host's clothing and infestations are associated with wearing the same clothing for prolonged periods of time without washing clothes (*e.g.*, wartime, natural disasters or poor personal hygiene). The Body Louse Genome Consortium (BLGC) proposed sequencing the human body louse genome (*3*). In the following article, we outline the rationale for sequencing this genome and the current status of the project along with critical issues that will be addressed with sequence information.

Biological Rationales for Sequencing the Body Louse Genome

Disease Transmission

Human body lice can be a serious public health threat as they transmit several types of bacteria that cause human diseases (*4*). The causative agent of body louse transmitted epidemic typhus is an obligatory intracellular alphaproteobacterium known as *Rickettsia prowazekii* (*5*) a category B bioterrorism agent (*6*, *7*). Symptoms of epidemic typhus include skin rashes, fever, chills, headaches, and exhaustion. Untreated cases of epidemic typhus, however, can be fatal. *R. prowazekii* also causes persistent chronic infection of humans that are interepidemic reservoirs. The disease is spread when the louse leaves febrile hosts with epidemic typhus. The louse itself eventually succumbs from rupture of the gut by growth of *R. prowazekii*, which then becomes available to infect a new host.

Prior to the development and wide-scale use of antibiotics, epidemic typhus was a major scourge of mankind, killing millions and having major impacts on military conflicts (*8*). Since the large-scale outbreaks of epidemic typhus in Europe through the mid 20th century, its occurrence has for the most part become sporadic (*9*). However, in 1986 more than 50,000 people in Burundi were infected and the disease has become re-emergent in other areas of the world (*2*). The agent is acquired by the lice from feeding on ill individuals, but is transmitted among humans primarily by aerosol and dermal inoculation of highly infected louse feces.

The spirochete *Borrelia recurrentis,* which is transmitted by the body louse, is closely related to the tick-borne relapsing fever species *B. duttonii* and is thought to have diverged from *B. duttonii* after its adaptation to the louse (*10*, *11*). In WWII, a million cases of louse-borne relapsing fever were observed in North Africa with a fatality rate of 10% (*2*). Lice feeding on *Borrelia*-containing blood become infected for life after the agent passes from the gut to the coelomic cavity. While lice cannot transmit the agent by feeding, the *Borrelia* readily penetrates skin or mucosal tissues if infected lice are crushed.

Bartonella quintana, a facultative intracellular alphaproteobacteria most closely related to *Brucella,* causes a five-day relapsing fever with long bone shooting pains and was responsible for more than a 1,000,000 cases in WWI on all European fronts (*2*). The agent is widespread in the homeless of developed countries and can cause persistent bacteremia and endocarditis and bacillary angiomatosis in HIV-positive individuals. Lice infected via blood meals remain persistently infected and *Bartonella* are excreted in large amounts from the intestine. Additionally, *Bartonella* can apparently be transmitted when the lice are feeding on their human hosts (*12*).

The genome sequences of *R. prowazekii* (*13*) and *B. quintana* (*14*), and *B. recurrentis* (*15*) have been determined as well as those of two species of *Borrelia* (*16*, *17*). Thus, determining the sequence of the body louse genome provides resources for expression arrays, reverse genetics for the molecular tools useful in the study of host-vector-bacterial pathogen interactions and provides a basis for genomic comparison with closely related species that do not transmit disease.

Smallest Known Genome Size for a Hemimetabolous Insect

The human body louse has the smallest genome known for any hemimetabolous insect (104.7 ± 1.4 Mb for females and 108.3 ± 1.1 Mb for males) (*18*). The recent sequencing of the body louse genome confirms its small size. In fact, the body louse genome is only slightly larger than that of *C. elegans* (100.4 Mb). For comparison, *Drosophila* genomes are 130-364 Mbp (*19*), the mosquito genomes of *Anopheles gambiae* and *Aedes aegypti* are 260 and 810 Mbp, respectively, and the ticks, *Ixodes scapularis* and *Boophilus microplus*, are 2,260 Mbp and 7,100 Mbp, respectively.

The Value of a Small Insect Genome, a Hemimetabolous Insect Genome, and a Parasitic Insect Genome

Lice are in the taxonomic group Paraneoptera (Acercaria or hemipteroid assemblage), which includes Hemiptera (true bugs, cicadas, whiteflies, leafhoppers, and aphids), Psocoptera (booklice, barklice, and psocids), Phthiraptera (lice), and Thysanoptera (thrips) (*20*, *21*, *22*). The other two hemimetabolous insects that will soon be completely sequenced are the pea aphid, *Acyrthosiphon pisum* (Aphididae), and the triatomid bug, *Rhodnius prolixus,* so the louse genome will assist in characterizing intraorder and interorder genetic changes in the Paraneoptera. The relationship of aphids, *Rhodnius,* and louse will provide critical comparative genomic tools to identify regions that are conserved among the Hemiptera (*e.g.*, exons and regulatory regions).

Lice are probably the most important single hemimetabolous group from the standpoint of human health. Many other hemimetabolous insects, nevertheless, have great impacts on the quality of life, including the migratory locust, aphids, bedbugs, and other pests. Additionally, the bloodsucking hemimetabolous insects may share significant novel bio-effector molecules not found in other arthropods of medical importance, such as ticks and mosquitoes. As such, the body louse sequence will provide important sources of genomic homology and contrast.

Parasites in general tend to have small genomes, yet the louse genome is exceptional even among these (*23*, *24*). Much as the relatively small fugu genome provides a contrast to the larger genomes of most other fish, the louse genome will show how insect genomes can be reduced (*25*, *26*, *27*).

Head Louse – a Close Relative of the Body Louse

Sequencing of the body louse genome will provide important insights into another major pest species, the human head louse. Head and body lice are so closely related that a long debate has occurred about whether they are subspecies or two separate species (*28*, *29*). The divergence of *Pediculus humanus* certainly occurred sometime after the divergence of chimpanzees and humans. The picture has become somewhat more complicated by the observation that there are two different populations of head lice which appear to have diverged between 0.77 and 1.18 million years ago and that body lice are more closely related to one of these lineages (*30*, *31*). The exact period when they diverged is not clear because the fossil record for lice is meager so that dating of molecular clocks is dependent on the accuracy of dating from the limited fossil hominid records, and estimates of the divergence of cercopithecoids and hominoids.

It has been suggested, however, that the origins of body lice occurred along with the origin of clothing and this occurred about 107,000 years ago (28). Body and head lice can mate and produce offspring, but their progeny are infertile, just like matings between horses and donkeys (32). Recent genetic evidence from double infestations of humans with both head and body lice has indicated that they are indeed two separate species (33). However, what we learn about the genome of body lice will likely provide us with important information in regards to head lice. This information may include, but certainly is not limited to, target sites (such as olfactory receptors) for the development of novel control agents. With modest additional funding, the current BLGC project could be extended to include sequencing of the head louse genome. If combined with the extensive EST libraries from head lice that now exist (Pittendrigh,

Clark, and Lee, unpublished data) sequencing efforts from these libraries should yield important insights into the differences between these two species.

Pediculosis

Pediculosis, caused by the human head louse, is the most prevalent parasitic infestation of humans in the United States. Lice are ubiquitous in most developing countries (2) and children 3 to12 yr old are most affected. Acquired immunity likely reduces louse density and impact on chronically exposed older juveniles and adults. Thus, louse outbreaks may constitute one of many opportunistic infections associated with a depressed immune system (*e.g.*, people with HIV). Unlike body lice, head lice have not been formally incriminated in the biological transmission of pathogens. However, it has been suggested that they may transmit *Rickettsia prowazekii* (34, 35) and head lice are known to mechanically transmit *Staphylococcus auereus* and *Streptococcus pyogenes* (36).

Although head louse infestations are irritating and can lead to infection, the social, mental, and economic consequences are even more substantial. Most people find head lice intolerable and often repeatedly and prophylactically apply costly pediculicides (insecticides) without realizing the potential harm and lethality if misused or overused. This impacts children in particular due to their small size and higher sensitivity to the toxic effects of these pediculicides (*37*).

Resistance to Traditional Control Methods

Treatment failures are common but the cause is uncertain (*e.g.*, resistance, improper application, misdiagnosis, formulation changes, etc.) (*38*). Nevertheless, louse resistance to most pediculicides is common and increasing in frequency (*2*, *39-57*), particularly to DDT, the pyrethrins and the pyrethroids. *Knockdown resistance* (*kdr*) is a major factor in all permethrin-resistant lice studied to date in the U.S. and supports the claim that treatment failure is, in part, due to resistance (*55*).

An observer-blind study on NIX® (Pfizer Consumer Healthcare, Morris Plains, NJ) (one percent permethrin crème rinse treatment) effectiveness validated these findings (*58*). In a recent survey of pharmacists, 78-82% of patients treated with synergized pyrethrins or permethrin remained infested and 63% treated themselves more often or at higher doses than mandated by the manufacturer (*59*). Predisposition of resistance to pyrethroids in DDT-resistant lice impacts current control measures that rely on natural pyrethrum or permethrin-amended shampoos. Thus, there is certainly a need for development of novel control agents for this pest.

U.S. pediculicide sales were last estimated as more than $150 million just for over-the-counter remedies. Infestation rates range from 6 to12 million cases annually. It is estimated that 2.6 million households are affected, with 8% of all school children infested (*2*). The overall cost of infestations is more than $367 million annually (*2*). The long-term impact of the days of lost learning by almost 1 in every 10 school-aged children due to the No-Nit policy and the lack of effective control options overshadows these cost estimates.

The pending loss of pyrethroids (*55*) and synergized pyrethrins (*43*) as effective pediculicides due to resistance is not trivial. Pyrethroids (*e.g.*, permethrin) are the safest and most effective class of insecticides available and are the principal choice for veterinary and medically important pests. Loss of control associated with resistance, however, has resulted in dangerous overuse (*60*, *61*, *62*, *63*). Incidences of injury and death increase as people resort to "home remedies," such as kerosene and gasoline. Without options, people overuse registered pediculicides, use combinations or resort to unregistered insecticides (*47*). Malathion (*e.g.*, Ovide®) is prescribed most often when pyrethroids fail. Malathion is one of the safest organophosphorous insecticides but is still an irreversible cholinesterase inhibitor. It causes a variety of chronic neuropathies, including organophosphate-induced delayed neuropathy, at near lethal dosages.

The current problems with louse control and resistance underscore the need to understand the molecular mechanisms of pesticide resistance in body and head lice. For example, the complete genome sequence for *Drosophila melanogaster*, which made possible the development of *Drosophila* oligonucleotide arrays with extensive gene coverage, has allowed researchers to determine a more complete complement of genes differentially expressed in pesticide-resistant strains of this species (*64*). Discovery of such resistance mechanisms can open up the possibility of using resistance-breaking compounds (*e.g.*, negative cross-resistance compounds) in novel manners to control pesticide-resistant populations (*65*, *66*).

Need for New Practices for Controlling Pediculosis

There are two ways to combat pediculosis: proactive prevention or post-infestation treatment. Emphasis is increasingly on prevention (education) and physical removal (combing or shaving) because a crisis exists in the chemical management of pediculosis. The pediculicide arsenal is limited and shrinking and health providers are spending an increasing and inordinate amount of time and resources dealing with infestations. Effective management information is lacking and few, if any, alternatives exist when standard pesticide treatments fail. Thus, there is a need for the discovery of new target sites in lice (such as olfactory receptors or genes for vitellogenin production) that could be used for the development of biocides that would selectively rid these pests of humans but not target humans. The genome project for body lice will hopefully provide the necessary core information to ultimately elucidate novel target sites for improved head and body lice control.

Understanding Genes Involved in Louse Behavior and Disease Transmission

Detection, treatment, and avoidance measures could be improved by gaining a greater understanding of molecular biology of how lice perceive the human body and head as a living habitat. The complete sequencing of the body louse genome has already opened the door to the development of cDNA or oligonucleotide arrays that can be used to gain a greater understanding of those genes that may be induced or repressed in lice in response to changes in their environment.

Body and head louse behavior could be altered and their populations reduced by exploiting target sites that impact the louse's behavioral patterns. For example, body lice exhibit a "homing instinct" towards their eggs (*67*, *68*) and feces (*69*), indicating that the response to ovipositional attractants is an important behavior that could be disrupted. The *Drosophila* genome project showed that olfactory receptors are species-specific and are represented by a diverse and rich set of gene families. Any and all of these could be targets for specific control. Similarly, vitellogenins or yolk proteins are formed only after a blood meal is taken in female mosquitoes and are probably also produced at high levels in blood fed mature lice as well (*70*). The protein-coding and regulatory regions of the genes involved in vitellogenesis, revealed by the sequencing effort, will also be potential target sites for control. Sequencing of the louse genome will also provide the scientific community with the knowledge to develop resources to understand the molecular mechanisms of disease transmission (*i.e.,* through the use of cDNA arrays or oligoarrays).

Chromosome Structure and Meiotic Failure

The centromere of the human chromosome remains an area of very active interest. Nondisjunction leading to polyploidy, monosomy and trisomy, remains the single largest contributor to infertility and mental retardation in man (*71*). Here the louse genome can make a unique contribution. Louse chromosomes are holocentric and behave as if the centromere is distributed throughout the genome. Male body lice also can exhibit both Mendelian and non-Mendelian inheritance of their paternal chromosomes but the environmental factors that contribute to this difference are unknown (*72*). A comparison of the louse genome to all other sequenced genomes, including that of humans, should provide fundamental information on the genomic basis of pairing and disjunction. Of potentially equal importance, male meiosis in the louse is achiasmatic, as is the case in *Drosophila* and in portions of the X and Y chromosomes of man. This would seem to be a parallel evolution, but it will be valuable to contrast the genomic basis of this process in different organisms.

Strategic Uses for the Sequence of the Body Louse Genome

The community of body louse investigators is relatively small, with about 50-200 scientists working on pediculosis and the biology of louse species. If, however, one extends this community to include those working on organisms that are more closely related to the louse than to any other sequenced genome (which includes aphids, *Rhodnius* and even ticks), this becomes a much larger community. Additionally, sequencing of the body louse genome will have broad implications for those considerably larger groups of researchers working on the disease organisms transmitted by body lice, and human researchers interested in the molecular biology of the body louse-human interactions. Moreover, the number of individuals that may be impacted by medical applications of improved pediculicides is considerable. The louse sequence will be important for those doing comparative genomics across insect taxa, as well as those interested in co-evolution of humans and their parasites.

A full genome sequence of the human body louse will now serve as the basis to begin to address health-related problems: (i) efficient discovery of target sites for potentially novel louse-specific biocides; (ii) discovery of genes involved in disease propagation and transmission; (iii) understanding of human-louse interactions; (iv) discovery of genes involved in attraction or repellency or both; and, (v) since there is relatively little information in the literature on the genomes of hemimetabolous insects when compared to holometabolous insects, this sequence will provide important information to those studying evolution of insect and other arthropod genomes.

Conclusions and Future Directions

The body louse genome represents one of the first hemimetabolous insect genomes to be completely sequenced and helps to fill a major gap in comparative genomics. Body lice can also be used as a model system to study how genomes are modified during an organism's adaptation to human parasitism.

With the complete genome sequence, the use of RNAi to knock out specific genes can be explored to identify genes responsible for allergens, insecticide resistance, host establishment, and pathogen transmission. Additionally, the availability to the scientific community of normalized body louse cDNA libraries, and a complete genome sequence, will facilitate the development of cDNA or oligonuocleotide arrays to: (i) discover new targets for the control of pediculosis, (ii) determine resistance mechanisms to current pediculicides, and (iii) identify physiological processes modified during infection by important and very diverse bacterial agents of human disease.

To this end, the Pittendrigh, Clark, and Lee laboratories have designed and created whole-genome oligonucleotide arrays from the body louse genome to begin to understand the molecular basis of pesticide resistance in head and body lice. In a preliminary proof-of-concept experiment, the transcriptional profiling of *P.h. humanus* genes induced by short-term exposure to sub-lethal concentrations to dexamethasone or ivermectin by microarray hybridization (Agilent Custom array with 8 x 15K format) was investigated.

Although we observed numerous candidate genes over-transcribed (88 for dexamethasone and 258 for ivermectin) and under-transcribed (190 for dexamethasone and 233 for ivermectin) due to these treatments (at $P<0.01$), of greatest importance are the following observations. Our initial results have revealed that dexamethasone caused over- and under-transcription of genes in the following groups: (i) cytochrome P450s (four for dexamethasone and eight for ivermectin), (ii) glutathione S transferases (none for dexamethasone and one for ivermectin), and (iii) esterases (two for dexamethasone and five for ivermectin). Additionally, both dexamethasone and ivermectin treatments caused over-and under-transcription of four different ABC transporter genes ($P<0.01$). We have initiated the process of performing quantitative real time PCRs to verify the over- and under-transcription of these candidate genes.

Acknowledgements

We thank K.Y. Mumcuoglu (Hebrew University, Jerusalem, Israel) for providing us the insecticide-susceptible human body louse colony maintained on rabbits. Funding Sources; National Pediculosis Association. "Large-scale Rearing of Head Lice." J.M. Clark, PI. ; NIH/NIAID (PHS 1 RO1 AI45062-01A1) "Detection of Insecticide Resistance in the Head Louse *Pediulus humanus capitis* and management of Pediculosis." J.M. Clark, P.I.; Indiana Center for Insect Genomics funds to BRP from Indiana 21st Century Fund. We also thank NHGRI/NIH for selecting the body louse for a genome-sequencing effort. NIX® is a registered trademark of Pfizer Consumer Healthcare, Morris Plains, NJ.

References

1. Pennisi, E. *Sci.* **2004,** 306, 210.
2. Raoult, D.; Roux, V. *Clin. Infect. Dis.* **1999,** 29, 888-911.
3. Pittendrigh, B. R.; Clark, J. M.; Johnston, J. S.; Lee, S. H.; Romero-Severson, J.; Dasch, G. A. *J. Med. Entomol.* **2006**, 43(6), 1103-1111.
4. Pan American Health Organization. *Proceedings of the International Symposium on the Control of Lice and Louse-Borne Diseases.* Scientific Publication No. 263. Pan American Health Organization, Washington, D.C.1973
5. Andersson, J. O.; Andersson, S. G. *Res. Microbiol.* **2000,** 151, 143-150.
6. Rotz, L. D.; Khan, A. S.; Lillibridge, S. R.; Ostroff, S. M.; Hughes, J. M. *Emerg. Infect. Dis.* **2002,** 8, 225-230.
7. Eremeeva, M. E.; Dasch, G.A. In *Encyclopedia of Bioterrorism Defense;* Pilch R. F.; Zilinskas R. A. Eds.; J. Wiley and Sons, Hoboken, NJ. 2005 pp 489-491.
8. Kelly, D. J.; Richards, A. L.; Temenak, J.; Strickman, D.; Dasch, G. A. *Clin. Infect. Dis.* **2002,** 34 (suppl. 4), S145-S169.

9. Weiss, K. In *Biology of Rickettsial Diseases*; D. H. Walker Ed.; CRC Press, Boca Raton, FL 1988; Vol. 1, pp. 1-14
10. Marti Ras, N.; La Scola, B.; Postic, D.; Cutler, S. J.; Rodhain, F.; Baranton, G.; Raoult, D. *Int. J. Syst. Bacteriol.* **1996,** 46, 859-865.
11. Cutler, S. J.; Moss, J.; Fukunaga, M.; Wright, D. J.; Fekade, D.; Warrell, D.; *Int. J. Syst. Bacteriol.* **1997,** 47, 958-968.
12. Kostrzewski, J. Bull. *Acad. Pol. Sci. Biol.* **1949,** 7, 233-263.
13. Andersson, S. G.; Zomorodipour, A.; Andersson, J. O.; Sicheritz-Ponten, T.; Alsmark, U. C.; Podowski, R. M.; Naslund, A. K.; Eriksson, A. S.; Winkler, H. H.; Kurland, C. G. *Nat.* **1998,** 396, 133-140.
14. Alsmark, C. M.; Frank, A. C.; Karlberg, E. O.; Legault, B. A.; Ardell, D. H.; Canback, B.; Eriksson, A. S.; Naslund, A. K.; Handley, S. A.; Huvet, M.; La Scola, B.; Holmberg, M.; Andersson, S. G. *Proc. Natl. Acad. Sci.* **2004,** 101, 9716-9721.
15. Lescot, M.; Audic, S.; Robert, C.; Nguyen, T. T.; Blanc, G.; Cutler, S. J.; Wincker, P.; Couloux, A.; Claverie, J. M.; Raoult, D.; Drancourt, M. *PLoS Genet.* **2008**, 4(9), e1000185.
16. Fraser, C. M.; S. Casjens, W. M.; Huang, G. G.; Sutton, R.; Clayton, R.; Lathigra, O.; White, et al. *Nature* **1997,** 390, 580-586.
17. Glockner G; Lehmann, R.; Romualdi, A.; Pradella, S.; Schulte-Spechtel, U.; Schilhabel, M.; Wilske, B.; Suhnel, J.; Platzer, M. *Nucleic Acids Res.* **2004,** 32, 6038-6046.
18. Johnston, J.S.; Yoon, K. S.; Strycharz, J. P.; Pittendrigh, B. R.; Marshall Clark, J. *J. Med. Entom.* **2007,** 44, 1009-1012.
19. Bosco, G.; Campbell, P.; Leiva-Neto, J. T.; Markow, T. A. *Genetics.* **2007**, 177(3), 1277-90.
20. Yoshizawa, K.; Johnson, K. P. *Mol. Phylogenet. Evol.* **2003,** 29, 102-114.
21. Murrell, A.; Barker, S. C. *Parasit. Res.* **2005,** 97, 274-280.
22. Yoshizawa, K.; Johnson, K. P. *Mol. Phylogenet. Evol.* **2005,** 37, 572-580.
23. Katinka, M. D.; Duprat, S.; Cornillot, E.; Metenier, G.; Thomarat, F.; Prensier, G.; Barbe, V.; et al. *Nat.* **2001**, 414, 450-453.
24. Sakharkar, K. R.; Dhar, P. K.; Chow, V. T. K. *Int. J. Syst. Evol. Microbiol.* **2004,** 54, 1937-1941.
25. Aparicio, S.; Chapman, J.; Stupka, E.; Putnam, N.; Chia, J. M.; Dehal, P.; Christoffels, A.; et al. *Sci.* **2002,** 297, 1301-1310.
26. Hedges, S. B.; Kumar, S. *Sci.* **2002,** 297, 1283-1285.
27. Venkatesh, B. In *Nature Encyclopedia of the Human Genome;* D.N. Cooper DN Ed., Vol. 2. Nature Publishing Group, London, UK. 2003 pp. 535-539.
28. Kittler, R.; Kayser, M.; Stoneking, M. *Curr. Biol.* **2003,** 13, 1414–1417.
29. Yong, Z.; Fournier, P. E.; Rydkina, E.; Raoult, D. *C. R. Biol.* **2003,** 326, 565–574.
30. Reed, D. L.; Smith, V. S.; Hammond, S. L.; Rogers, A. R.; Clayton, D. H.; *PLoS Biol.* **2004,** 2, e340.
31. Leo, N. P.; Barker, S.C.; *Parasitol. Res.* **2005,** 98, 44-47.
32. Ferris, G. F. *Pacific Coast Entomol. Soc. Mem.* **1951,** 320.

33. Leo, N. P.; Campbell, N. J. H.; Yang, X.; Mumcuolglu, K.; Barker, S.C. *J. Med. Entomol.* **2002,** 39, 662–666.
34. Goldberger, J. *Publ. Hlth. Rep.* **1912,** 27, 297-307.
35. Murray, E. S.; Torrey, S.B. *Ann. NY Acad. Sci.* **1975,** 266, 25-34.
36. Meinking, T. L. *Curr. Prob. Dermatol.* **1999,** 11, 73-120.
37. National Research Council. *Pesticides in the diets and of infants and children.* National Academy Press, Washington D.C.1993;
38. Pollack, R. J.; Kiszewski, A.; Armstrong, P.; Hahn, C.; Wolfe, N.; Rahman, H. A.; Laserson, K.; Telford III, S. R.; Spielman, A. *Arch. Pediatr. Adolesc. Med.* **1999,** 153, 969-973.
39. Hurlbut, H. S.; Altman, R. M.; Nibley, C. Jr. *Sci.* **1952,** 115, 11-12.
40. Cole, M. M.; Couch, M. D.; Burden, G. S.; Gilbert, I. H. *J. Econ. Entomol.***1957,** 50, 556-559.
41. Wright, J. W.; Brown, A. W. A. *Bull. WHO* **1957,** 16, 9-31.
42. Wright, J. W.; Pal, R. *Bull. WHO* **1965,** 33, 485-501.
43. Cole, M. M.; Clark, P. H. *J. Econ. Entomol.* **1961,** 54, 649-651.
44. Clark, P. H.; Cole, M. M. *J. Econ. Entomol.* **1964,** 57, 205-210.
45. Clark, P. H.; Cole. M. M. *J. Econ. Entomol.* **1967,** 60, 398-400.
46. Miller, R. N.; Wisseman, C. L.; Sweeney, G. W.; Verschueren, A.; Fabrikant, I. B. *Amer. J. Trop. Med. Hyg.* **1972,** 66, 372-375.
47. Blommers, L.; Van Lennep, M. *Entomol. Exp. App.* **1978,** 23, 243-251.
48. Maunder, J. W. *J. Roy. Soc. Hlth.* **1991,** 24-26.
49. Chosidow, O.; Chastang, C.; Brue, C.; Bouvet, E.; Izri, M.; Monteny, N.; Bastuji-Garin, S.; Rousset, J. J.; Revuz, J. *Lancet* **1994.** 344, 1724-1727.
50. Mumcuoglu, K. Y.; Hemingway, J.; Miller, J.; Ioffe-Uspensky, I.; Klaus, S.; Ben-Ishai, F.; Galun, R. *Med.Vet. Entomol.* **1995,** 9, 427-432.
51. Rupes, V.; Moravec, J.; Chmela, J.; Ledvinka, J.; Zelenkova, J. *Centr. Eur. Publ. Hlth.* **1995,** 3, 30-32.
52. Gratz, N. G. *Human lice: their prevalence, control and resistance to insecticides.* World Health Organization, Switzerland. 1997.
53. Picollo, M. I.; Vassena, C. V.; Casadio, A. A.; Massimo, J.; Zerba, E. N. *J. Med. Entomol.* **1998,** 35, 814-817.
54. Downs, A. M. R.; Stafford, K. A.; Coles, G. C. *Parasitol. Today.* **1999,** 15, 1-4.
55. Lee, S. H.; Yoon, K. S.; Williamson, M. S.; Goodson, S. J.; Takano-Lee, M.; Edman, J. D.; Devonshire, A.; Clark, J. M. *Pestic. Biochem. Physiol.* **2000,** 66, 130-143.
56. Meinking, T. L.; Entzel, P.; Villar, M. E.; Vicaria, M.; Lemard, G. A.; Porcelain, S. L. *Arch. Dermatol.* **2001,** 137, 287-292.
57. Meinking, T. L.; Serrano, L.; Hard, B.; Entzel, P.; Lemard, G.; Rivera, E.; Villar, M. E. *Arch. Dermatol.* **2002,** 138, 220-224.
58. Meinking, T. L. C.; Chen, C. M.; Kolber, M. A.; Tipping, R. W.; Furtek, C. I.; Villar, M. E.; Guzzo, C. A. *J. Pediatr.* **2002,** 141, 665-670.
59. Pray, W.; Hosp, S. *Pharm.* **2003,** 38, 241-246.
60. Aldridge, W. N. In *Pyrethroid Insecticides: Chemistry and Action* J. Mattieu Ed., Ronde Rouseel UCLAF, Romainville, France, 1980; Vol. 37 pp. 45-47.

61. LeQuesne, P. M.; Maxwell, I. C.; Butterworth, S. T. G. *Neurotoxicol.* **1980,** 2, 1-11.
62. Rose, G. P.; Dewar, A. *J. Arch. Toxicol.* **1983,** 53, 297-316.
63. Kaloyanova, F. P.; El Batawi M. A. *Human Toxicology of Pesticides.* CRC Press, Boca Raton, Florida. 1991.
64. Pedra, J. H. F.; McIntyre, L. M.; Scharf, M. E.; Pittendrigh, B. R. *Proc. Nat. Acad. Sci.* USA. **2004,** 101, 7034-7039.
65. Pedra, J. H. F.; Hostetler, A.; Gaffney, P. J.; Reenan, R. A.; Pittendrigh, B. R. *Pestic. Biochem. Physiol.* **2004,** 78, 58-66.
66. Pittendrigh, B. R.; Gaffney, P. J.; Huesing, J. E.; Onstad, D. W.; Roush, R. T.; Murdock, L. L. *J. Theor. Biol.* **2004,** 231(4), 461-74.
67. Bacot, A. *Parasitol.* **1917,** 9, 228-258.
68. Nuttall, G. H. F. *Parasitol.* **1917,** 10, 5-185.
69. Wigglesworth, V. B. *Parasitol.* **1941,** 33, 67-109.
70. Attardo, G. M., II.; Hansen, A.; Raikhel, A. S. *Insect Biochem. Mol. Biol.* **2005,** 35, 661-675.
71. Hassold, T.; Hunt, P. *Nat. Rev. Genet.* **2001,** 2, 280-91.
72. McMeniman, C. J.; Barker, S. C. *Heredity.* **2006,** 96, 63-68.

Chapter 15

Resistance Management of the Human Head Louse Using Molecular Tools

Si Hyeock Lee[1], J. Marshall Clark[2], Kyong Sup Yoon[2], Deok Ho Kwon[1], Hilliary E. Hodgdon[2] and Gun Mook Seong[1]

[1]Department of Agricultural Biotechnology, Seoul National University, Seoul, Korea 151-742
[2]Department of Veterinary & Animal Sciences, University of Massachusetts, Amherst, MA 01003

Head lice resistance to permethrin is mainly conferred by the knockdown resistance (*kdr*) trait, a voltage-sensitive sodium channel (VSSC) insensitivity factor. Three VSSC mutations have been identified and confirmed to reduce the sensitivity of VSSC to permethrin. A step-wise resistance monitoring system has been established based on molecular resistance detection techniques. Quantitative sequencing (QS) has been developed to predict the *kdr* allele frequency in head lice at a population basis. The speed, simplicity and accuracy of QS made it an ideal candidate for a routine primary resistance monitoring tool to screen a large number of wild louse populations as an alternative to conventional bioassay. As a secondary monitoring method, real-time PASA (rtPASA) has been devised for more precise determination of low resistance allele frequencies. To obtain more detailed information on resistance allele zygosity, as well as allele frequency, serial invasive signal amplification reaction (SISAR) has been developed as an individual genotyping method. Our approach of using three tiers of molecular resistance detection should facilitate large-scale routine resistance monitoring of permethrin resistance in head lice using field-collected samples.

The pyrethrins, pyrethroids and malathion are the major commercially available pediculicides in the current market. Extensive use of the pyrethrins/pyrethroids as over-the-counter pediculicides, however, was rapidly followed by resistance. Pyrethroid resistance in head louse populations appears to be widespread both in the United States and other countries but varies in intensity and is not yet uniform *(1)*. Thus, establishment of proactive resistance management system is essential to maximize the life span of these major pediculicides prior to the complete fixation of head lice resistance. Loss of these valuable pediculicides in the current market due to the development of resistance would cause a serious problem in the control of pediculosis.

Detection of the early phase of resistance is crucial to the long-term, efficient resistance management that can delay and reverse the resistance development. However, early resistance detection is very difficult using conventional bioassay-based monitoring methods, particularly when resistance is recessive. In addition, collecting large numbers of live specimens, particularly in case of lice, is often impractical and always difficult. To circumvent these limitations, various individual genotyping techniques for the detection of resistance allele frequencies using genomic DNA extracted from target insects have been employed as alternative resistance monitoring tools *(2,3)*. For the efficient monitoring of head lice resistance in the field based on resistant genotype, we have developed a tire of molecular tools, including quantitative sequencing (QS), real-time PCR amplification of specific allele (rtPASA) and serial invasive signal amplification reaction (SISAR). In this chapter, we describe and compare the features of individual techniques and how to employ them in routine resistance monitoring of head lice that is practical and cost-efficient.

Molecular detection of head louse resistance to pyrethrins and pyrethroids

QS

Three point mutations (M815I, T917I and L920F) in the voltage-sensitive sodium channel (VSSC) α-subunit gene have been determined to be responsible for permethrin resistance of head lice *(4-6)*. QS was developed as a population genotyping method for the prediction of the VSSC mutation frequencies in head lice on a population basis *(7)*. Detailed procedures of QS are described elsewhere *(7)*. In brief, a 908-bp genomic DNA fragment of the VSSC α-subunit gene, encompassing the three mutation sites (M815I, T917I and L920F), was PCR-amplified from individual genomic DNAs. Individual PCR products from susceptible and resistant head lice were sequenced to confirm the genotypes at each mutation site and to identify any sequence polymorphisms in the intron regions. Once the genotypes and the intron sequences were confirmed, the PCR products with or without mutations were mixed to generate the standard DNA mixture templates in following molar ratios: 0:10, 1:9, 3:7, 5:5, 7:3, 9:1 and 10:0 (resistant allele : susceptible allele at each mutation site). Standard DNA template mixtures (10 ng) were sequenced with an ABI prism 3730 DNA sequence analyzer (Applied Biosystem, Foster City, CA) using Big Dye Terminator cycle sequencing kit (Applied Biosystem) and two sets of sequencing primers for the sense- and antisense-directional sequencing, respectively (NICEM Sequencing Facility, Seoul National University, Korea). The nucleotide signal intensities of the resistant and susceptible alleles at each mutation site were determined from the sequence chromatogram using Chromas Ver 2.31 software (Technelysium Pty Ltd., Tewantin, AUS) and the signal ratios were calculated using following equation 1.

Equation 1

$$\text{Signal ratio} = \frac{\text{Resistant nucleotide signal}}{\text{Resistant nucleotide signal} + \text{Susceptible nucleotide signal}}$$

Individual DNA templates from heterozygous lice were also sequenced as an internal reference to the 5:5 standard DNA template. The signal ratios of template DNA mixtures were normalized by multiplying them with the normalization factor (signal ratio of the heterozygous DNA template/signal ratio of the 5:5 standard DNA template). The series of normalized signal ratios were plotted against the corresponding resistance allele frequencies, and standard regression equations together with lower and upper prediction equations were generated using the SIGMA plot ver 10.0 (Systat Software Inc., San Jose, CA) for the estimation of resistance allele frequencies of unknown samples and their prediction intervals at the 95% confidence level.

When a set of standard DNA mixtures with different ratios of resistant and susceptible alleles were sequenced, the signal intensity of each resistant nucleotide increased as the resistance allele frequency increased (Fig. 1A). When nucleotide signal ratios at the M915I mutation locus were plotted against the corresponding resistance allele frequencies at each mutation site and fitted to quadratic equations (Fig. 1B), the resulting regression curves showed high correlation coefficients (r^2 = 0.9928~0.9997), demonstrating that the nucleotide signal ratio is highly proportional to the resistance allele frequencies. Since the correlation coefficients usually varied slightly, depending on the sequencing direction, and result in different prediction equations at each mutation site (data not shown), regression equations with both higher regression coefficients and narrower prediction intervals can be chosen for the prediction of mutation frequency. Similar results were also obtained with other two mutations (data not shown).

Using the lower and upper 95% prediction equations, the M815I mutation allele frequencies could be accurately predicted within the range of 9.7~90.9% at the 95% confidence level *(7)*. Likewise, the lower detection limits for other two mutations (T917I and L920F mutations) were determined as 8.0% and 4.4% at the 95% confidence level, respectively. In summary, the lower detection limits for the three resistance mutations were 4.4~9.7% (7.4 ± 2.7%), suggesting that QS can be employed as a preliminary resistance monitoring tool for the detection of resistance allele frequencies higher than ca. 7.4% at the 95% confidence level *(7)*.

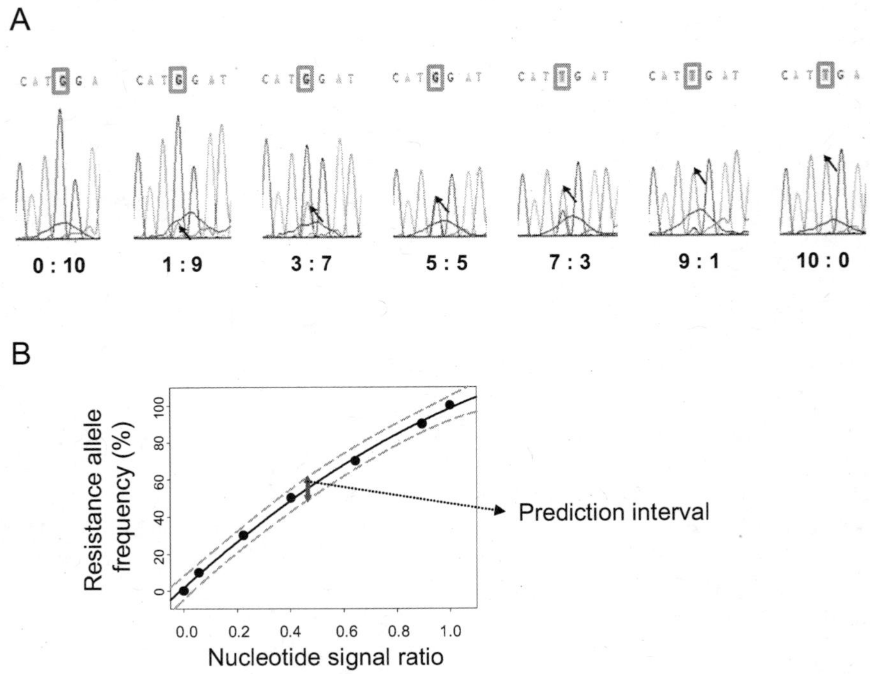

Figure 1. Sequencing chromatograms of the standard template DNA mixtures with different ratios of resistant and susceptible alleles (A) and the plot of resistance sequence signal ratio versus resistance allele frequency at the M815I mutation site (B). The relative intensities of the resistance allele signals are indicated with arrows in Panel A. Quadratic regression line is indicated by a solid line with the upper and lower 95% prediction lines indicated by dotted lines in Panel B.
(See page 3 of color inserts.)

Changes in the DNA template quantity for QS did not affect the plot properties, indicating that template amount is not a critical factor in QS performance as long as nucleotide signal ratio is used for constructing the plots. The same set of standard DNA templates repetitively generated virtually the same regression equations as long as an identical sequencing instrument is used for QS. Once established, therefore, a set of standard regression and prediction equations can be repetitively used for the prediction of allele frequencies of unknown samples without sequencing the standard DNA templates each time.

When resistance allele frequencies in several head louse populations were predicted by QS and compared with those determined by individual sequencing, the actual resistance allele frequency of each population was included within the 95% prediction interval generated by QS, demonstrating the reliability and accuracy of QS in predicting resistance allele frequency *(7)*. The resistance allele frequency in a louse population mostly composed of heterozygous individuals was also precisely estimated by QS. Presence of phenotypically susceptible heterozygous lice in a field population would not be detected by a traditional bioassay due to the recessive trait of the knockdown resistance (*kdr*) factor *(8)*, emphasizing the importance of DNA-based detection of resistance allele frequency and zygosity in resistance monitoring.

There were no significant differences in predicted allele frequencies between the 'pooled DNA' (DNA extracted from individual louse specimens, then combined and prepared) and 'pooled specimen DNA' (DNA extracted and prepared from multiple louse specimens all at once) as long as the size (developmental stage) and quality (collected and stored in the same way) of individual lice are identical. This finding validates our approach of using the 'pooled specimen DNA' as the DNA template for QS-based population genotyping. 'Pooled specimen DNA' prepared from louse specimens of mixed stage (i.e., different size) cannot be used for QS because the variation in DNA quantity among individual lice would result in misrepresentation of resistant allele frequency in the combined population. Nevertheless, the use of DNA extracted from combined multiple lice for QS greatly reduces the overall cost and effort as repetitive DNA extraction from individual lice is arduous and costly.

Resistance allele frequencies at the three mutations were virtually identical as determined by QS, corroborating that the three mutations exist together in a resistant haplotype in the head louse. If this is always the case, resistance allele frequency can be predicted using any of the three mutations. Since the T917I mutation alone plays a crucial role in permethrin resistance by making the sodium channel virtually insensitive to the action of permethrin *(6)*, QS-based prediction of allele frequency can be conducted using only this to save time and resources. Since the reliable lower detection limit for resistance allele frequency prediction by QS is ca. 7.4% (approximately equivalent to the population with one homozygous resistant individual out of 14 louse specimens or one heterozygous resistant individual out of 7 louse specimens), QS with small to medium-size populations (for example, 14-28 louse specimens per population) appears adequate and a practical approach for routine population genotyping.

The T929I mutation frequencies in head louse populations from different geographical regions were analyzed by QS (Fig. 2). Resistance allele frequencies varied substantially in lice from different global regions. Resistance allele frequencies are completely saturated or near saturation in lice from South Florida (USA), Onkaparinga (Australia), Bristol (UK), and Bobigny (France) as judged by the predicted frequencies near 100%. Lice from California and Texas appear to be moderately resistant to pyrethroid as judged by their mean resistance allele frequencies (86.2% and 60.4%, respectively). The predicted resistance allele frequency was 5.2% in lice from Ecuador and 1.5% in lice from Guatemala and Thailand. These findings confirm our original contention that permethrin resistance in head lice is currently wide spread but not uniform *(1)*. Resistance alleles appear more prevalent in developed countries, which may be due to the more extensive use of pyrethrin/pyrethroid-containing pediculicides in these countries.

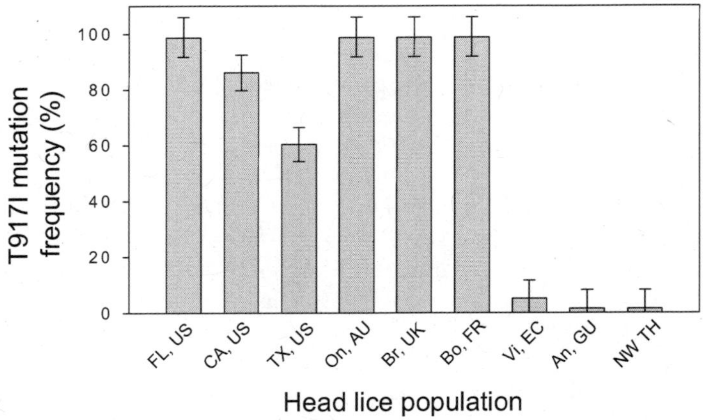

Figure 2*. Resistance allele frequencies of lice from different global locations at the T917I mutation site predicted by QS population genotyping method. Error bars indicate upper and lower prediction interval at the 95% confidence level. Louse populations were collected from following regions: FL, US (Plantation & Homestead, FL, USA); CA, US (San Bernadino County, CA, US); TX, US (Jefferson & Orange Counties, TX, US); On, AU (Onkaparinga, Australia); Br, UK (Bristol, UK); Bo, FR (Bobigny, France); Vi, EC (Vilcabamba, Ecuador); An, GU (Antigua, Guatemala); NW TH (Northwestern Thailand)*

rtPASA

The rtPASA protocol was developed to detect the resistance allele frequencies below the lower detection limit of QS (ca. 7.4%). The same 908-bp genomic DNA fragment of the VSSC α-subunit gene, used as the template for QS, was PCR-amplified and used for rtPASA. The standard DNA mixture templates for rtPASA were prepared by combining the PCR-amplified fragments with and without the M815I, T917I and L920F mutations in following ratios: 0:100, 1:99, 3:97, 8:92, 16:84 (resistant allele : susceptible allele at each mutation site). Resistant allele-specific primers were designed to match the I917 and F920 alleles simultaneously whereas susceptible allele-specific primers to match T917 and L920 alleles simultaneously (Fig. 3). Real-time PCR (rtPCR) with allele-specific primers (each 5 pM) and standard DNA mixture template (1 ng) was conducted using the Chromo 4^{TM} real-time thermal cycler (Bio-Rad, Hercules, CA). Following rtPCR, threshold cycles (Ct) were determined from each amplification curve, normalized to the Ct value of 0% resistant allele frequency, and plotted against respective resistance allele frequencies. Standard linear regression lines were generated by plotting the log of the resistant allele frequency versus Ct value using the SIGMA plot ver 10.0 (Systat Software Inc.). The PCR amplification efficiency (E) was calculated from the slope of the standard curve using the following equation: $E=10^{-1/slope}$.

The optimum conditions for the rtPASA were determined to be 64℃ annealing temperature, 5 pM each primer, 1 ng DNA template. Based on the relationship between resistance allele frequencies (0~16%) and corresponding Ct values (Fig. 4A), a linear regression line (y=-3.24x + 10.32, r^2=0.999) was generated by converting the frequency to log values (Fig. 4B). The high regression coefficient demonstrated a very strong correlation between resistance

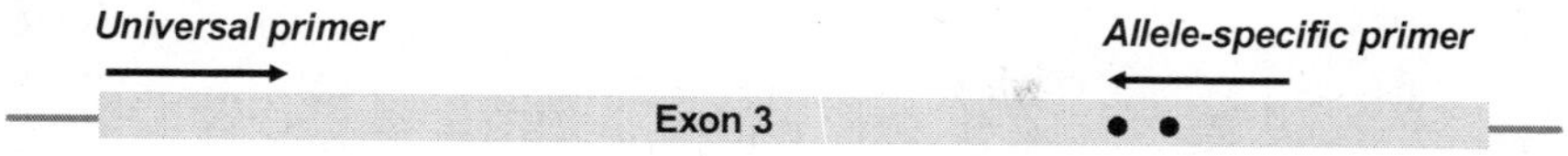

Figure 3. *Diagram of the exon 3 fragment in the VSSC genomic DNA region that encompasses the T917I and L920F mutation sites. Locations of the two mutations are marked with black circles. Horizontal arrows indicate the locations of the rtPASA primers.*

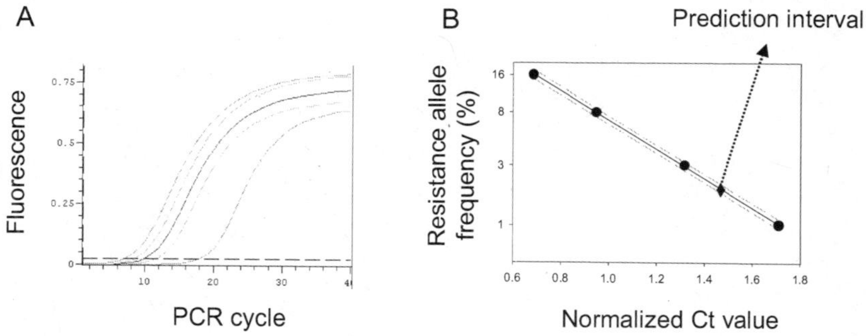

Figure 4. *Typical amplification patterns of rtPASA using the DNA templates containing 0~16% resistant alleles (A) and the regression line generated from the plot of normalized Ct value versus the log of resistance allele frequency (B). The regression line is indicated by a solid line with the upper and lower 95% prediction lines indicated by dotted lines in Panel B (See page 4 of color inserts.).*

allele frequency and Ct value. The resistance allele frequency of 1% was clearly distinguishable from 0% but those lower than 1% (i.e., 0.3% and 0.1%) were not distinguishable, indicating that the lower detection limit for rtPASA is around 1%. Considering the prediction interval, the lower detection limit was determined as 1.13% at the 95% confidence level.

Genomic DNA samples extracted from the head louse populations collected from Ecuador, Thailand and Korea were analyzed by rtPASA. The resulting Ct values from the regional lice DNA samples were converted to actual allele frequencies using the equation generated by the set of the standard DNA mixtures. The resistance allele frequencies in the Ecuador, Thailand and Korea populations were estimated as 8.0%, 0%, and 16.2%, which corroborated well with those determined by QS (5.2%, 1.5% and 11.7%, Fig. 2).

SISAR

The SISAR technology, based on a fluorescence resonance energy transfer (FRET) detection format, has been developed for the high throughput detection of single nucleotide polymorphisms (SNPs) *(9)* using structure-specific endonucleolytic cleavage by eubacterial DNA polymerases *(10)*. This high throughput genotyping method detects sodium channel mutations associated with permethrin resistance in individual head lice *(11)*. Detailed protocols, including the sequences of FRET cassettes, invasive and probe oligonucleotides, are well described elsewhere *(11)*. Briefly, a 1.1-kb VSSC genomic DNA fragment containing the M815I, T917I and L920F mutation sites was amplified by PCR, serially diluted, and heat-denatured at 95°C for 10 min. The denatured DNA from individual samples or synthesized target DNAs for control reactions were added to individual wells on the pre-dried SISAR microplate with SISAR reagents, and incubated at four different temperatures (60.5, 63.5, 66.5, or 69.5°C) using a PTC-200 Thermal Cycler (MJ Research, Waltham, MA). Relative fluorescent units (RFU) from the SISAR samples were determined using the Gemini XS fluorescent spectrophotometer (Molecular Dynamics, La Jolla, CA) at 1 h intervals for the duration of the assay. Fluorescence for the susceptible and resistant nucleotides was determined by using fluorescein and Cy3, respectively. Net fold-over-zero (Net-FOZ) for each dye and the SISAR ratio were determined according to the manufacture's instruction and are given in Equations 2 and 3, respectively.

Equation 2

$$\text{Net-FOZ} = \frac{\text{RFU from probe (resistant or susceptible)}}{\text{RFU from no target control}} - 1$$

Equation 3

$$\text{SISAR ratio} = \text{Net FOZ resistant} / \text{Net FOZ susceptible}$$

The genotypes of 27 individual head lice, collected from Mathis, TX, US, were analyzed by employing the optimized SISAR protocols, and compared with those determined by direct DNA sequencing. All SISAR kits for each mutation discriminated the genotypes with 100% accuracy. The frequencies of the resistant homozygous, heterozygous and susceptible homozygous alleles were determined as 11.1%, 51.9%, and 37.0%, respectively, resulting in the total resistant allele frequency of 37.1% (Fig. 5).

The individual genotyping based on SISAR is very accurate and efficient in obtaining detailed information on resistance allele frequency and allelic zygosity. However, since SISAR requires relatively a large number of samples to ensure accurate estimation of resistance allele frequency, it is more suitable for the secondary or tertiary resistance monitoring step.

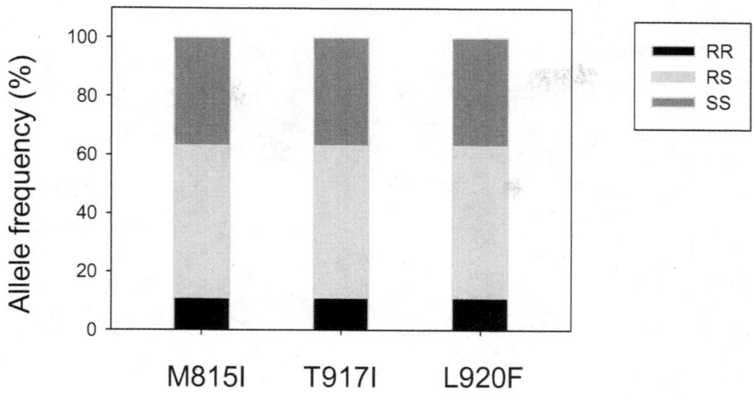

Figure 5. Estimation of resistant allele zygosity and frequency by SISAR at the three VSSC mutation sites of a head louse population collected from Mathis, TX, US.

Head louse resistance management

Three molecular methods for head lice resistance detection were compared using the criteria of technical dependency, reliability, sensitivity, zygosity detection, cost, time, suggested usage in resistance monitoring and suggested number of lice per analysis (Table I). QS-based population genotyping can process a large number of louse populations simultaneously for the evaluation of resistance allele frequencies. It is expected that QS of 90 different population samples can be completed within 2 days in moderately equipped laboratories (1 day for genomic DNA extraction, 3 hrs for PCR to generate DNA templates for QS, and 5 hrs for sequencing). The technique dependency of QS is also relatively low compared to other population genotyping techniques such as rtPASA-TaqMan *(12)* and rtPASA. Thus, the speed, simplicity and moderate sensitivity of QS make it an ideal candidate for a routine primary resistance monitoring tool to screen a large number of wild louse populations as an alternative to conventional bioassay. Since the sensitivity of QS is ca. 7.4%, a small to medium-size sampling (7~14 lice) per louse population should be sufficient, making this method practical considering the difficulty of collecting a large number of lice samples.

Taken together, prediction of resistance allele frequency by QS will greatly facilitate the initial resistance monitoring efforts in field populations of lice. The QS-based population genotyping protocol should be readily applicable for other insects, including other human louse species as long as information on resistance-associated mutations exists.

Table I. Comparison of molecular techniques for resistance detection.

	QS	rtPASA	SISAR
Technical dependency	Low	Moderate	Low
Reliability	High	High	Very high
Sensitivity (Detection limit for resistance allele frequency)	Moderate (7.4%)	High (1.12%)	Can detect actual frequency
Zygosity detection	No	No	Yes
Cost per sample[a]	$2.0	$1.5	$1.5
Time per 96 samples[b]	2 days	2 days	2 days
High throughput analysis	Yes	Yes	Yes
Suggested usage in resistance monitoring	Primary	Secondary	Secondary or tertiary
Suggested no. of lice per analysis for resistance monitoring	7~14	50~100	50~100

[a] Costs include DNA extraction and PCR. The cost for QS and rtPASA is for analyzing a single population as a unit whereas the cost of SISAR for analyzing a single individual as a unit.

[b] The time includes DNA extraction and PCR. The time for QS and rtPASA is for analyzing 90 populations plus 6 standard DNA templates whereas the time for SISAR for 96 individuals.

If more precise determination of resistance allele frequency below the QS detection limit is required on a population basis, rtPASA can be employed as a supporting monitoring step. This method enabled the detection of the *kdr* allele frequency in the head lice at the level as low as 1.13%. To detect the resistance allele frequencies lower than ca. 1%, however, a large-size sampling (50~100 lice per population) would be required. In addition, the technical dependency of rtPASA is relatively high, requiring a well optimized protocol and experimental system to ensure an accurate prediction.

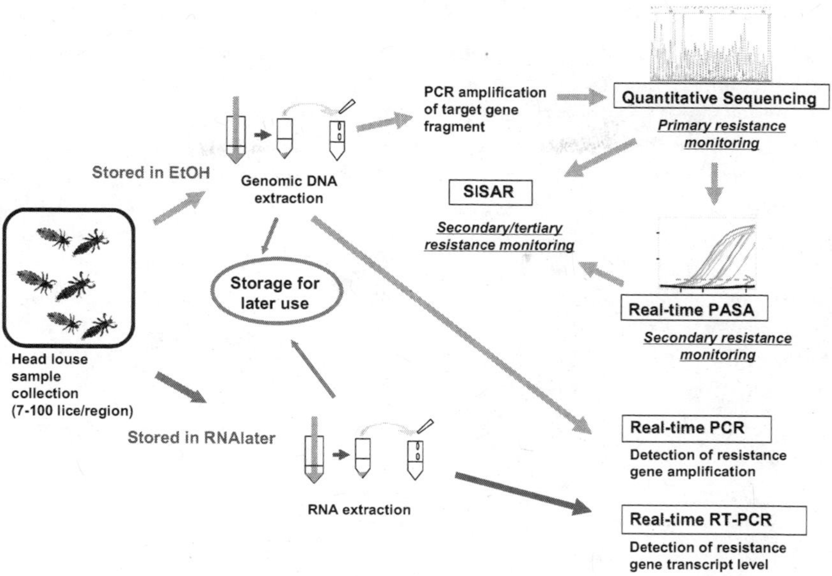

***Figure 6**. Schematic diagram of head lice resistance monitoring tire using several molecular tools.*
(See page 4 of color inserts.)

Although both QS and rtPASA enable the prediction of resistance allele frequencies on a population basis, thereby allowing rapid screening of resistant populations, they do not provide information on allele zygosity. If the information on resistance allele zygosity as well as allele frequency in a population is required, individual genotyping methods such as SISAR *(11)* can be conducted on a much reduced number of preselected populations as the secondary or tertiary resistance monitoring step. Information on allele zygosity would be particularly useful for understanding the resistance population dynamics at the early phase of resistance. SISAR requires, however, a large number of analyses (50~100 analyses of individual lice per population) to ensure accurate estimation of resistance allele frequency, which limits its applicability for a primary routine resistance monitoring tool.

Taken together, the three molecular tools discussed in this chapter can be readily employed for routine resistance monitoring of head louse populations in a tire system as shown in Fig. 6. In this scheme, DNA samples are extracted from a batch of louse specimens and processed for primary and secondary/tertiary resistance monitoring steps. If possible, RNA also can be extracted and stored for later use possibly in the real-time quantitative PCR for transcription profiling of over- or under-expressed genes putatively associated with resistance. If the resistance allele is less than approximately 7% when judged by QS (close to the detection limit of QS), the population can be examined using a second tier method such as rtPASA or SISAR. DNA samples are also useful in copy number determinations of duplicated genes putatively associated with resistance and in population genetic studies for investigating the resistance dynamics based on DNA markers including microsatellite dinucleotide repeats *(13)*. In addition to detecting permethrin resistance mediated by *kdr* trait, a major factor in all permethrin-resistant lice worldwide *(4)*, accumulation of yearly and regional database on resistance allele frequencies will greatly facilitate the monitoring and understanding of resistance evolution patterns in different geographical regions over time. Based on the resistance allele frequencies estimated by these molecular techniques, differential actions for resistance management should be invented. In regions where resistance allele frequency is saturated or near saturation, pyrethroids use should be curtailed and alternative pediculicides with different mode of actions used instead. In regions where the resistance allele frequencies are low or near zero, pyrethroids should be used cautiously and in conjunction with resistance monitoring program. This approach will extend the effective life span for this valuable group of pediculicides.

Acknowledgements

This work was supported by the NIH/NIAID (R01 AI045062-04A3). D. H. Kwon and G. M. Seong were supported in part by the Brain Korea 21 Program.

References

1. Gao, J.-R.; Yoon, K. S.; Lee, S. H.; Takano-Lee, M.; Edman, J. D.; Meinking, T. L.; Taplin, D.; Clark, J. M. *Pestic. Biochem. Physiol.* **2003**, *77*, 115-124.
2. Clark, J. M.; Lee, S. H.; Kim, H. J.; Yoon, K. S.; Zhang, A. *Pest Manag. Sci.* **2001**, *57*, 968974-7.
3. Kim, H. J.; Hawthorne, D. J.; Peters, T.; Dively, G. P.; Clark, J. M. *Pectic. Biochem. Physiol.* **2005**, *81*, 85-96.
4. Lee, S. H.; Yoon, K. S.; Williamson, M. S.; Goodson, S. J.; Takano-Lee, M.; Edman, J. D.; Devonshire, A. L.; Clark, J. M. *Pestic. Biochem. Physiol.* **2000**, *66*, 130-143.
5. Lee, S. H.; Gao, J.-R.; Yoon, K. S.; Mumcuoglu, K. Y.; Taplin, D.; Edman, J. D.; Takano-Lee, M.; Clark, J. M. *Pestic. Biochem. Physiol.* **2003**, *75*, 79-91.
6. Yoon, K. S.; Symington, S. B.; Lee, S. H.; Soderlund, D. M.; Clark, J. M. *Insect Biochem. Mol. Biol.* **2008**, *38*, 296-306.
7. Kwon, D. H.; Yoon, K. S.; Strycharz, J. P.; Clark, J. M.; Lee, S. H. *J. Med. Entomol.* **2008**, *(in press)*.
8. Yoon, K. S.; Gao, J.-R.; Lee, S. H.; Clark, J. M.; Brown, L.; Taplin, D. *Arch. Dermatol.* **2003**, *139*, 994-1000.
9. Hall, J. G.; Eis, P. S.; Law, S. M.; Reynaldo, L. P.; Prudent, J. R.; Marshall, D. J.; Allawi, H. T.; Mast, A. L.; Dahlberg, J. E.; Kwiatkowski, R. W.; de Arruda, M.; Neri, B. P.; Lyamichev, V. I. *Proc. Natl. Acad. Sci. USA* **2000**, *97*, 8272-8277.

10. Lyamichev, V.; Brow, M. A.; Dahlberg, J. E. *Science* **1993**, *260*, 778-783.
11. Kim, H. J.; Symington, S. B.; Lee, S. H.; Clark, J. M. *Pestic Biochem Physiol* **2004**, *80*, 173-182.
12. Livak, K. J. *Genet Anal* **1999**, *14*, 143-149.
13. Leo, N. P.; Hughes, J. M.; Yang, X.; Poudel, S. K.; Brogdon, W. G.; Barker, S. C. *Heredity* **2005**, *95*, 34-40.

Chapter 16

Monitoring of *kdr*-Mediated Pyrethroid Resistance in Head Louse Colonies in Japan

Shinji Kasai[1], Norihisa Ishii[2], Masaru Natsuaki[3], Hiroyuki Fukutomi[4], Osamu Komagata[1], Mutsuo Kobayashi[1] and Takashi Tomita[1]

[1]Department of Medical Entomology, National Institute of Infectious Diseases,
1-23-1 Toyama, Shinjuku-ku, Tokyo 162-8640, Japan
[2]Department of Bioregulation, Leprosy Research Center,
National Institute of Infectious Diseases,
4-2-1 Aoba-cho, Higashimurayama-shi, Tokyo 189-0002, Japan
[3]Department of Dermatology, Hyogo College of Medicine,
1-1 Mukogawa-cho, Nishinomiya, Hyogo 663-8501, Japan
[4]SMS Corporation, 541-2 Tsuruma, Machida-shi, Tokyo 194-0004, Japan

Recently, in Japan, cases of head louse infestation have been gradually increasing and this increase is a social concern. Phenothrin, the only registered active ingredient used as a pediculicide in Japan has been in use since 1981. Development of insecticide resistance within Japanese head lice colonies has been suspected as the main factor in the reemergence of head lice infestations in this country. Therefore, we investigated the current level of insecticide resistance in the head louse population in Japan. We focused on the four resistance-associated amino acid substitution mutations in the *para*-orthologous sodium channel gene, which is the target site of pyrethroids and 1,1,1-trichloro-2,2-bis(4-chlorophenyl)ethane (DDT). Head lice were collected through the efforts of dermatologists, public health centers, and our departmental website. DNA was extracted from each larva, adult, or nit and the frequency of four mutations were monitored using a genotyping assay. Overall, 282 head louse colonies were collected from 22 prefectures in Japan. Nineteen louse colonies contained knock down resistance *(kdr)* -like sodium channel mutations and the frequency of occurrence of resistant colonies was 6.7%. Resistant head lice were confirmed in 10 prefectures. We could not determine if development of insecticide resistance is the main factor in the recent increase in head lice infestations in Japan. However, based on results from other countries, the occurrence of *kdr*-type head louse colonies is expected to increase. Thus, it is necessary to prepare alternative louse control agents.

Introduction

Pediculosis, caused by the head louse (*Pediculus capitis* De Geer) is a human ectoparasitic disease that is becoming a world wide social concern. The number of head louse cases in Japan had been collected by the Ministry of Health and Welfare (Japan) from 1981 until data collection was discontinued in 1999. We combined those Japan national data with that from the Tokyo metropolitan area collected from 1995 to 2007 (Figure 1). The 1995 to 1999 trends in the numbers of reported cases between the two statistic sources were similar, and based on the order of magnitude difference between the two data sources. Moreover, we expect the current approximate number of cases in Japan to be 10 times the Tokyo metropolitan value (Figure 1).

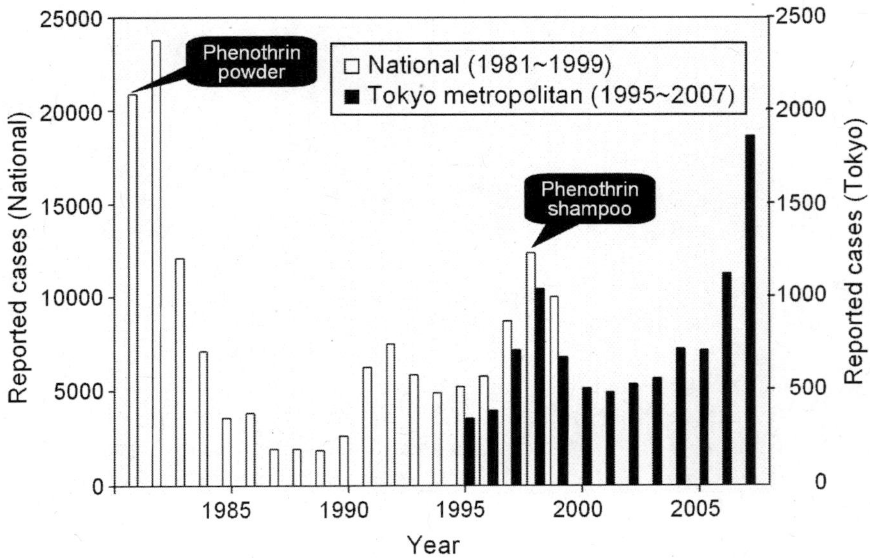

Figure 1. *Annual number of head louse cases in Japan. (National data,1981–1999, left vertical axis; Tokyo metropolitan data, 1995–2007, right vertical axis).*

There was a marked peak in head louse infestation in the early 1980s. A pediculicide, Sumithrin® powder, containing the pyrethroid phenothrin as the active ingredient, was placed on the Japanese market in 1981. Subsequently, the number of reported head louse cases decreased markedly over the next several years. The number of pediculocis, however, gradually increased from the beginning of 1990's. Although the number of reported cases temporarily decreased by the appearance of more convenient Sumithrin® shampoo, also containing phenothrin as the active ingredient, in 1998, pediculosis cases are again increasing in the last several years (Figure 1).

We hypothesized three reasons for the recent reemergence of pediculosis in Japan. First, life style changes could be involved as the number of parents taking predominant care of their children is decreasing and the chances of children contacting other children while camping or at day care facilities, kindergarten, or school are increasing. Secondly, we speculated that the number of infested people in, or coming back into, Japan is increasing due to recent increases in international travel. Third, we suspected that development of insecticide resistance might have resulted in pediculicide failure. Phenothrin is the only active ingredient of pediculicide in the Japanese market and more than one half million of Sumithrin® shampoos/powders are used annually in Japan. Thus, we investigated the phenothrin susceptibility of head lice collected in Japan.

Emergence of phenothrin resistant head louse colonies in Japan

It is difficult to obtain a sufficient number of head lice samples from a human host and to use dosage-knockdown regression analysis which is usually applied for insect bioassays. In addition, head lice, once removed from the human head, are relatively weak as compared to body lice (1). Thus, louse survival longevity is short, resulting in high control mortalities. Therefore, we established a rapid evaluation method to determine phenothrin susceptibility in head louse (2). Using this method, 15 living head louse colonies collected in the Tokyo metropolitan area in 2001 and 2002, were assayed. Of those 15, 3 colonies, designated as R1, R2, and R3, were judged to be resistant to phenothrin. This was the first evidence of phenothrin resistant head louse colonies in Japan (3).

Sequencing full length of *para* sodium channel cDNA

We sequenced whole cDNA of the *para* sodium channel, which is the reported target site of pyrethroid insecticides and DDT (4). The full length cDNA consisting of 6261 bp encoded 2086 amino acid residues (4). The sodium channel from the head louse exhibited the high similarities to that from the German cockroach *Blattella germanica* (90% positional identity), *Drosophila melanogaster* (88%), and the house fly *Musca domestica* (86%) in a joined partial alignment window with 1021 amino acid positions corresponding to domains I to IV, but excluding the three inter-domain-linking segments and the N- and C-terminal inner cellular domains. The cDNA sequences of the sodium channel from phenothrin-susceptible and -resistant head lice colonies were compared. Although three independent resistant colonies were analyzed, all three shared the same cDNA sequences. As a result, 24 nucleotide differences between susceptible and resistant colonies were confirmed. Among them, only 4 nucleotides resulted in amino acid substitutions: D11E in the N-terminal inner-membrane segment, M815T in the outer-membrane loop between the *trans*-membrane segments four and five of domain II, and T929I and L932F in the *trans*-membrane segment five of domain II (Figure 2). The latter two substitutions have been reported from pyrethroid-resistant head lice collected from the USA and the UK (5).

Recently, an electrophysiological study revealed that three of the abovementioned point mutations (i.e., M815I, T929I, and L932F) are associated with pyrethroid resistance in head louse (6). All combinations of these mutations were inserted into the sodium channel gene of housefly and expressed in *Xenopus* oocytes. Their experiments revealed that each of the three mutations resulted in a reduction in permethrin sensitivity and the T929I mutation, which has been functionally validated as a *kdr*-like mutation in diamondback moth *Plutella xylostella* (7), was the primary cause of resistance development.

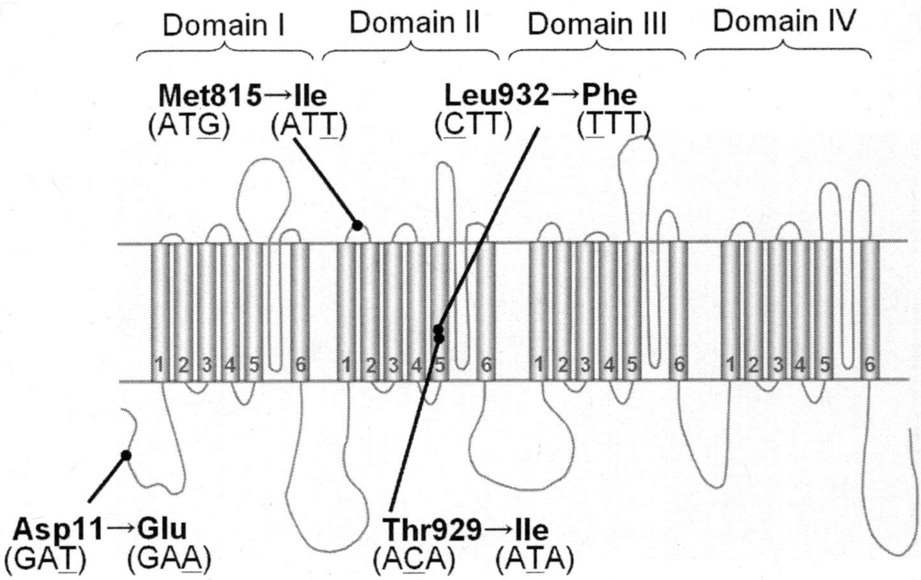

Figure 2. *Four amino acid substitutions found in the para sodium channel of phenothrin-resistant head louse colonies*

Use of a genotyping method to simultaneously target four mutations

In order to investigate the frequency of *kdr*-like alleles in the head louse colonies collected in Japan, we established a genotyping method to simultaneously target the four abovementioned mutations in each individual head louse (8). We collected head louse samples via dermatologist mailing lists, a departmental web page advertising the project, and members of medical entomology and zoology societies in Japan. In the departmental website, we included a questionnaire asking for information on the host children, including gender, age, history of phenothrin usage, and email address if the provider wanted to know the analysis result. Shortly after analysis, the result was reported to the sample provider. Avoidance or termination of phenothrin treatment was recommended to the sample provider if a *kdr*-like allele was detected. From December 2006 to March 2008, we collected 630 head lice from 282 infested people, of which approximately 80 percent were female. This female predominance may be related to the hair of young females being relatively longer than those of males, thus making it easier to catch head louse from other children during close encounters. Host age composition is shown in Figure 3. Six and seven year old children were most common, and more than 96% of the hosts were less than 13 years old (Figure 3).

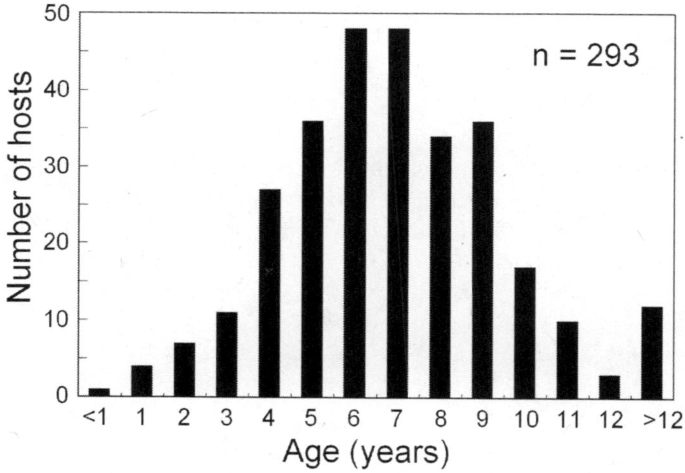

Figure 3. *Age composition of the head louse hosts*

Among the 630 head lice tested, 55 lice homozygously or heterozygously possessed *kdr*-like genes. The ratio of RR:RS:SS was 47:8:575 (R and S represent resistant and susceptible alleles, respectively). The frequency of occurrence of resistant genes in the total individuals was 8.7% (55/630). The number of colonies which possessed at least one *kdr*-like allele was 6.7% (19/281). Notably, all four mutations existed concomitantly in the *kdr*-like alleles. Since the same haplotype was confirmed in a strain of resistant head louse in Florida, USA (9), it is probable that *kdr*-type resistance in head louse is induced by a single haplotype of the sodium channel gene worldwide. The head louse samples were collected from 22 prefectures in Japan and *kdr*-like alleles were confirmed in the lice collected from 11 prefectures (Figure 4). These results indicate that resistant head lice are distributed extensively throughout Japan.

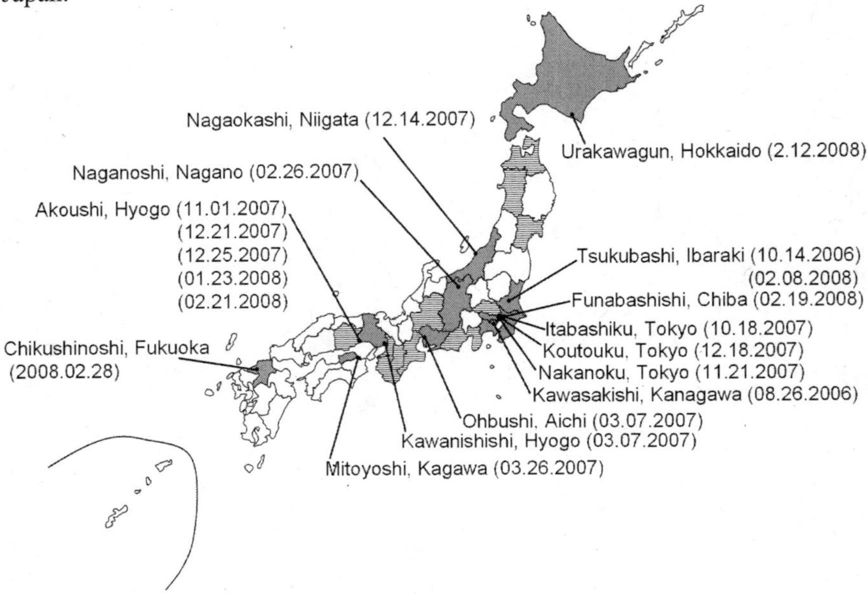

Figure 4. *Geographical distribution of resistant head louse in Japan. Sample collection dates for prefectures with resistant head louse are indicated in parenthesis. Regions with horizontal lines indicate prefectures where sample(s) were collected but no kdr-like allele was detected.*

Conclusions

As shown in Figure 5, the frequencies of *kdr*-like alleles are high in several developed countries, including the USA, Denmark, and the UK (10-12). The values exceeded more than 90%, especially in the USA (Florida) and Denmark. This suggests that pyrethroid insecticides are not effective in those areas. On the contrary, the frequency of *kdr*-like alleles in Japan remains less than 10% so that pyrethroids would still be effective against most head louse populations. Phenothrin has been used as a pediculicide in Japan for nearly 30 years. Low frequency of the *kdr*-like allele in Japan is probably due to comparatively recent migration of the resistant individual(s) from abroad. However, it is expected that the prevalence of resistant head lice will increase annually and reach a high percentage in near future because more than one half million of Sumithrin® shampoos/powders are used annually in Japan; thus producing a significant amount of phenothrin resistance selection pressure. In Japan, phenothrin is the only active ingredient registered for head louse control. We suggest that educational facilities, including kindergartens, nursery schools, and elementary schools, will see increased head louse infestations if phenothrin loses its effectiveness against head lice. This indicates that new pediculicides need to be registered and placed on the market as soon as possible. Lately, new active ingredients, such as dimeticone and isopropyl myristate have been developed and are becoming popular in other countries, including Canada and the UK. These compounds are non-neurotoxins, originally developed as cosmetic components, and have a physical action on lice that may not result in resistance development (13, 14). It has also been reported that these compounds have almost the same effectiveness against head lice as pyrethroids (13, 14). Introduction of these compounds to Japan is desired. In the meantime, monitoring of the relative abundance of *kdr*-like alleles in Japan needs to be continued, at least until new pediculicides are widely available.

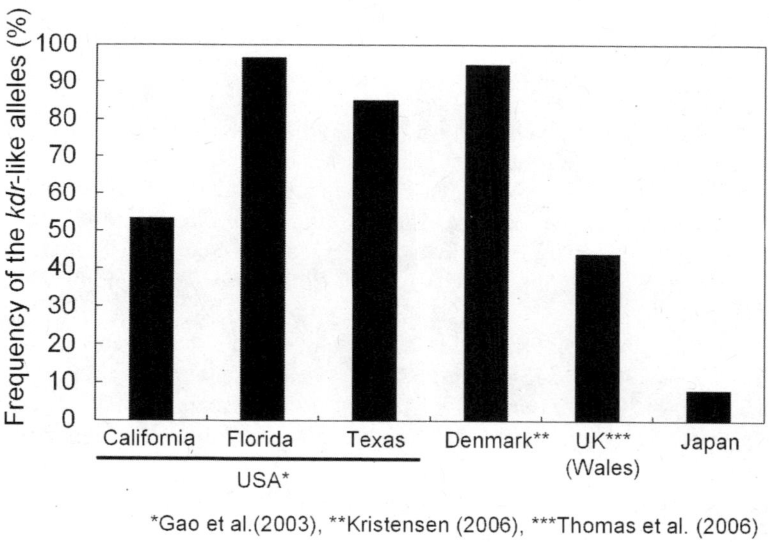

Figure 5. *Prevalences of kdr-like alleles in the USA, Denmark, the UK, and Japan*

*Data of *, **, and *** are cited from references (10), (11), and (12), respectively.*

Acknowledgments

The authors thank all collaborators who kindly provided head louse samples. This work was partially supported by a Grant-in-Aid for Scientific Research on Emerging and Re-emerging Infectious Diseases from the Ministry of Health, Labour and Welfare, Japan (H18-Shinko-Ippan-009).

References

1. Mihara, M. *Life and Sci.* **1999**, 44, 23-32.
2. Kasai, S.; Mihara, M.; Takahashi, M.; Agui, N.; Tomita, T. *Med. Entomol. Zool.* **2003**, 54, 31-36.
3. Tomita, T.; Yaguchi, N.; Mihara, M.; Agui, N.; Kasai, S. In *Environmental Fate and Safety Management of Agrochemicals*, Clark, J. M.; Ohkawa, H. eds., **2005**, Vol. 899, pp. 234-243. Washington, D.C., American Chemical Society
4. Tomita, T.; Yaguchi, N.; Mihara, M.; Takahashi, M.; Agui, N.; Kasai, S. *J. Med. Entomol.* **2003**, 40, 468-474.
5. Lee, S. H.; Ingles, P. J.; Williamson, M. S.; Goodson, S. J.; Takano-Lee, M.; Edman, J. D.; Devonshire, A. L.; Clark, J. M. *Pestic. Biochem. Physiol.* **2000**, 66, 130-143.
6. Yoon, K. H.; Symington, S. B.; Lee, S. H.; Soderlund, D. M.; Clark, J. M. *Insect Biochem. Mol. Biol.* **2008**, 38, 296-306.
7. Schuler, T. H.; Martinez-Torres, D.; Thompson, A. J.; Denholm, I.; Devonshire, A. L.; Duce, I. R.; Williamson, M. S. *Pestic. Biochem. Physiol.* **1998**, 59, 169-182.
8. Kasai, S.; Ishii, N.; Natsuaki, M.; Fukutomi, H.; Komagata, O.; Kobayashi, M.; Tomita, T. *J. Med. Entomol.* (in press)
9. Lee, S. H.; Gao, J. R.; Yoon, K. S.; Mumcuoglu, K. Y.; Taplin, D.; Edman, J. D.; Takano, L. M.; Clark, J. M. *Pestic. Biochem. Physiol.* **2003**, 75, 79-91.
10. Gao, J. R.; Yoon, K. H.; Lee, S. H.; Takano-Lee, M.; Edman, J. D.; Meinking, T. L.; Taplin, D.; Clark, J. M. *Pestic. Biochem. Physiol.* **2003**, 77, 115-124.
11. Kristensen, M.; Knorr, M.; Rasmussen, A.-M.; Jespersen, J. *J. Med. Entomol.* **2006**, 43, 533-538.
12. Thomas, D. R.; McCaroll, L.; Roberts, R.; Karunaratne, P.; Roberts, C.; Casey, D.; Morgan, S.; Touhig, K.; Morgan, J.; Collins, F.; Hemingway, J. *Arch. Dis Child.* **2006**, 91, 777-778.
13. Burgess, I. F.; Brown, C. M.; Lee, P. N. *BMJ* **2005**, 330, 1423.
14. Kaul, N.; Palma, K. G.; Silagy, S. S.; Goodman, J. J.; Toole, J. *J. Cutan. Med. Surg.* **2007**, 11, 161-167.

Indexes

Author Index

Subject Index

D

E

F

G

H

I

M

N

O

P